Nursing and HIV/AIDS

The printing of this document was made possible
by a grant to the American Nurses Foundation
from Becton Dickinson and Company.

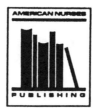

American Nurses Publishing is the publishing program
of the American Nurses Foundation, an affiliate organization
of the American Nurses Association.

c.

The American Nurses Association (ANA) and the ANA HIV Task Force thank all of the individuals and groups who have supported nursing's efforts in the area of HIV/AIDS care. Our special thanks to Becton Dickinson and Company; Cliff Morrison, M.S.N., R.N., F.A.A.N.; Helen Schietinger, M.A., R.N., M.F.C.C.; and all whose writing, review, and comments contributed to the publication of this document.

HIV Task Force, 1992-1994
Barbara Russell, M.P.H., R.N., C.I.C., B.S.H.A., Chairperson
Joanne Deutsche, R.N., C.
Allen Harris, B.S.N., R.N., C.
Deborah Coleman, M.S., R.N., C.S.
Barbara Aranda-Naranjo, M.S., R.N.
Cecil King, C.N.O.R., R.N.
Sarah Stanley, M.S., R.N., C.N.A., C.S., Senior Policy Analyst, ANA
Valarie Carty, Administrative Assistant, ANA

HIV Matrix Team
Colleen Scanlon, J.D., R.N., Director, Center for Ethics and Human Rights, ANA
Winifred Carson, J.D., Practice Counsel, ANA
Deborah McNeal Arrindell, Associate Director, Department of Governmental
    Affairs, ANA
Barbara Sapin, Labor Counsel, ANA
Karen Worthington, M.S., B.S., R.N., Staff Specialist, Labor Relations, ANA

ISBN 1-55810-097-0

Published by American Nurses Publishing
600 Maryland Avenue, SW
Suite 100 West
Washington, DC 20024-2571

CONTENTS

iii

PREFACE

The American Nurses Association's (ANA) first publication to describe the care of persons with HIV/AIDS, *Nursing and HIV: A Response to the Problem* (ANA 1988), helped outline the issues of the pandemic in the 1980s. *Nursing and HIV/AIDS* provides an update of the issues with a clear nursing focus, and supplements existing resources that describe the clinical issues associated with HIV/AIDS. This publication is designed for nurses involved in direct practice, education, administration, research, and/or health policy, as well as for nursing students.

Definitions of the scope of nursing practice and the nature of nursing that are used in this document are taken from *The Scope of Nursing Practice* (ANA 1987) and *Nursing: A Social Policy Statement* (ANA 1980). ANA's Social Policy Statement describes the nature of nursing as complex and highly interactive, and asserts that society has historically understood nursing to be a non-invasive, nurturing discipline focused on creating the type of physiological, psychological, and sociocultural environment in which people with HIV/AIDS can gain or maintain health.

This publication was developed using the nursing functions of care, coordination, education, advocacy, and research. All of these functions include consideration of the physical, psychosocial, spiritual, ethical, legal, and political issues involved in the prevention of illness, promotion of health, and coordination of care for persons with HIV/AIDS. New knowledge concerning clinical, epidemiological, statistical, and work force issues develops almost daily; nurses are therefore encouraged to contact the Centers for Disease Control and Prevention (CDC) and professional nursing or other health care organizations for the most current scientific information about HIV infection.

ANA and ANA's HIV Task Force hope that *Nursing and* HIV/AIDS will enhance the abilities of both the individual nurse and the nursing profession to respond to the HIV pandemic with competency and compassion.

INTRODUCTION

Acquired immunodeficiency syndrome (AIDS) has profoundly affected our society, wreaking devastation on personal lives and communities. Successfully responding to those infected with the human immunodeficiency virus (HIV) and preventing further transmission will be dependent on our society's values and sense of community. In the early 1980s, nursing's orientation to the needs of persons with HIV/AIDS was demonstrated by the many nurses who provided direct patient care and developed comprehensive and innovative models of care for persons with HIV infection.

The HIV/AIDS pandemic is not the first widespread disease outbreak for which nurses have been challenged to provide care. Nurses have historically provided distinctive skills and leadership in response to numerous health care challenges.

Nurses distinguished for their courage during various pandemics include:

- Florence Nightingale, who worked in Scutari during the Crimean War, from 1854 to 1856;
- Lillian D. Wald and Lavinia Lloyd Dock, who during 1892 and 1893 provided nursing services to the immigrants of New York City;
- Jane Delano, who worked prior to and during World War I in the United States and in Europe; and
- Clara Louise Maas, who provided nursing care during the yellow fever pandemic in Cuba.

Countless other nurses have cared for the sick in other pandemics—such as influenza, poliomyelitis, tuberculosis, and syphilis. Nursing has always provided leadership in illness and care, health promotion, the organization of care, and research.

Nursing uniquely focuses on human responses (occurring throughout the life span) to alterations in function as a consequence of genetic, physiological, cognitive, emotional, social, and environmental changes. The human responses to HIV/AIDS include those of the individual who has symptoms of HIV infection, who has been exposed to the virus, or who is concerned about potential exposure, as well as those of the individual's partner, family, and/or community.

The concerns and needs of persons with HIV infection, their families (biological or chosen), and their friends are as numerous, varied, and complex as their individual circumstances. Confrontation with a progressive, debilitating, fatal illness creates profound stress and suffering. Therefore, the unique skills and expertise of the nurse in providing care, coordination, education, and advocacy to meet the challenges of fatal diseases are essential in addressing the human and scientific challenges posed by HIV. Such expertise includes helping the person with HIV infection to maintain optimal quality of life.

The future course of the HIV pandemic is uncertain because a vaccine or curative therapy does not yet appear to be on the horizon. Although we do know how to stop further transmission of HIV, the ways in which this information is disseminated must be reexamined. For example, information on preventing transmission has not been readily available in some instances, and the information that has been available often has not been easily accessible to individuals who do not speak English or who have limited facility with written language.

Providing the necessary information in a format effective enough to promote behavior changes requires more than newspaper or magazine articles, brochures, lectures, conferences, or informational meetings. Halting further HIV transmission requires much more—values clarification and an understanding of life styles that may be markedly different from one's own.

Our society is at a critical juncture. Policies determined during this period of mobilization for prevention and control of the disease will affect both nurses and their patients. The needs of society, as well as of the individual person with HIV/AIDS, mandate that nurses be involved in setting policy on this issue. The full nursing community—including nurses providing direct patient care, nurse administrators, nurse educators, and state and national nursing coalitions/organizations—must continue to be concerned and involved.

Effective responses to HIV/AIDS will be determined by the members of society whose education, skills, and practice provide them with the knowledge essential for strong leadership. In collaboration with other disciplines within the health care system, and through community outreach efforts, nursing can and must provide the leadership necessary to meet the multifaceted challenges associated with the HIV/AIDS pandemic.

Epidemiology

Overview

The first cases of the disease eventually classified as HIV/AIDS were reported to the Centers for Disease Control and Prevention in 1981 (Centers for Disease Control 1981a, 1981b). The etiological agent, a retrovirus, was not isolated until 1983 (Institute of Medicine 1986; von Reyn and Mann 1987). Since that time, the human immunodeficiency virus has been recognized as the cause of one of the most significant health crises of the 20th century.

The CDC developed a definition of AIDS for surveillance purposes in 1982. Since then, as a result of increasing knowledge about the disease, the definition has been revised several times (see Appendix C). All cases that meet this definition are required to be reported to local health departments, which in turn report aggregate numbers and demographic data to the CDC. HIV/AIDS is a pandemic, affecting all inhabited countries and continents throughout the world. AIDS cases have been officially reported to the World Health Organization (WHO) by 164 countries, and HIV infection has been documented in virtually all countries (Mann, Tarantola, and Netter, 1992).

In the United States, 315,390 cases of HIV/AIDS were reported to the CDC between 1981 and 1993 (Centers for Disease Control 1993b). More than 50 percent of these people have died. Based on current trends, the CDC projects that the number of living people diagnosed with AIDS according to the 1987 case definition will have increased from approximately 90,000 in 1992 to approximately 120,000 by January 1995 (Centers for Disease Control 1993b).

HIV/AIDS accounts for an increasing percentage of total mortality in the United States. While mortality rates from most other leading causes of death decline or remain relatively stable, the death rate from HIV/AIDS continues to climb. In 1991, HIV/AIDS was the ninth leading cause of death among all age groups and the third leading cause of death among persons 25 years to 44 years of age (Centers for Disease Control 1993a). The increasing role of HIV as a cause of death among men and women in this age group has a disproportionately severe impact on society as a result of the loss of otherwise productive years of life, and the loss of parents from families with young children.

As acknowledged by the CDC, estimating the total number of HIV-infected persons remains a complex and inexact task. In 1988, for example, public health experts estimated the number of HIV-infected persons in the United States to be anywhere from 800,000 to 1,200,000, of which more than 50 percent did not know they were infected, and the majority of which did not perceive themselves as having HIV/AIDS (U.S. Public Health Service 1988).

After HIV was discovered to be the cause of AIDS, highly sensitive and specific HIV antibody tests became available, the spectrum of manifestations of HIV infection became better defined, and classification systems for HIV infection were developed (Centers for Disease Control 1992; Haverkos et al. 1985; Redfield, Wright, and Tramant 1986). (The CDC's 1993 revised HIV classification system is presented in Appendix C.)

AIDS occurs at the end stage of HIV disease and is the most severe manifestation of HIV infection. As the natural history of HIV is studied, more is learned about the disease process in various demographic populations. By 1990, it became obvious that some progressive, seriously disabling, and even fatal conditions (e.g., encephalopathy, wasting syndrome) affecting a substantial number of HIV-infected patients were not subject to epidemiologic surveillance since they were not included in the AIDS case definition.

In collaboration with public health and clinical specialists, the CDC responded by developing the most recent revision of the case definition for surveillance (CDC 1992), which includes the CD4 T-lymphocyte count and the addition of three conditions (disease caused by M. *tuberculosis*, recurrence [two or more episodes within a year] of pneumonia or invasive cervical cancer). The new definition is intended to reflect the clinical reality and current understanding of the disease more effectively, and increases the number of reported cases by including either:

1. the diagnosis of an opportunistic infection or malignancy that is indicative of immune suppression, with no underlying reason for the immunosuppression, or
2. a positive HIV antibody test and a CD4 T-lymphocyte count of less than 200 cells per microliter of blood.

Natural History

Each year, more is understood about the natural history of HIV disease and the factors associated with rapid disease progression. Two indicators—the time from infection with HIV to the onset of AIDS, and the time from the diagnosis of AIDS to death—have been examined extensively among various populations. In one study of homosexual men, 50 percent developed AIDS within 9.2 years from the date of HIV infection (Hendrik et al. 1993). In a study of hemophiliacs, 45 percent developed AIDS within 12 years from the date of HIV infection (Sabin et al. 1993).

On a large scale, these indicators are useful tools, both for evaluating the effectiveness of new therapies and for anticipating the need for HIV-related health and social services. On an individual level, this information is useful for making treatment decisions and for estimating a person's potential length of life. However, there is a complex set of factors affecting these indicators, and one must use caution when making general statements about an individual's prognosis or survival time based on this information. Disease progression and survival time differ markedly according to demographic characteristics, the availability of appropriate medical care, and the use of improved therapies for treatment and prophylaxis. Further, these indicators will be affected by the 1992 revision to the AIDS case definition for surveillance (CDC 1992).

Nurses must be aware of the "window period"—the time from exposure to evidence of HIV antibodies (0 to 6 months). This is not to be confused with the "incubation period," which can be as long as 10 years. Individuals may not know they are incubating the disease until symptoms of the disease appear or until they are tested.

The time from infection to onset of AIDS (*incubation period*) and the time from diagnosis of AIDS to death (*survival time*) differ according to clinical characteristics such as CD4 counts, the presence of an AIDS-indicating condition, and the type of AIDS-defining illness (Hanson et al. 1993; Pratt et al. 1993).

These clinical characteristics can differ according to the demographics of the population being studied. For instance, age is independently related to survival as measured by the indicators, with individuals over 45 years and infants having a poorer prognosis than young adults (Turner et al. 1993). In one study of perinatally infected children, the median survival time was 9.2 years (Pratt et al. 1993). In a study of adult transfusion-related AIDS cases, the median survival time in the 13- to 40-year-old group was 273 days, compared to 58 days in the 41- to 64-year-old group, and 60 days in the group aged 65 years and over (Sutin et al. 1993).

In various studies, the indicators differ according to race, gender, and modes of transmission, but these differences have been shown to be related to underlying differences in socioeconomic factors among the various groups studied (Bastian et al. 1993; Curtis and Patrick 1993). An analysis of nine studies of survival time found that the studies which minimized socioeconomic differences between Caucasians and African Americans showed no significant difference in survival time by race, while studies that did not account for socioeconomic differences seemed to indicate significantly shorter survival times for African Americans (Curtis and Patrick 1993).

Routes of Transmission

Epidemiologic studies confirm that AIDS is not transmitted through casual contact (Gershon, Vlahov, and Nelson 1990). Since the early 1980s, routes of HIV transmission have been recognized as sexual (anal, vaginal, and, to a lesser degree, oral contact), parenteral (involving the sharing of needles, mainly for intravenous injections but also for other injectable routes), and perinatal (recent prospective studies suggest that the risk of perinatal transmission is likely to be 30 percent or less [Boland and Conviser 1992]). Blood, semen, and vaginal secretions are the three body fluids documented to be involved in HIV transmission. Other possible transmission could occur from the presence of blood in another body substance.

Individuals at the highest risk for HIV infection include men having sex with men, injection drug users who share needles, women having sex with infected men, infants born to infected women, and, to a lesser degree, men having sex with infected women. Those at lower risk include women having sex with women, individuals who have received blood products, and health care workers who experience significant exposure to the blood of an HIV-infected individual through injury with a sharp instrument. Potentially risky procedures/activities that could cause HIV transmission through infected blood include organ/tissue transplants, tattooing, and the use of contaminated instruments or shared personal hygiene implements.

First Decade Changes in the Epidemiology

The epidemiology of HIV has gradually changed over the first decade of the pandemic. While the numbers of cases have continued to rise steadily among all transmission categories, the incidence of AIDS has increased in some and leveled off in others. The percentage of women infected through heterosexual transmission has persistently increased. The geographic concentration of the disease in urban inner cities continues, except for a climb in cases in the rural South.

Since the beginning of the pandemic, the largest number of HIV/AIDS cases has been in the transmission category of men having sex with men. Now, however, the incidence of HIV/AIDS among gay and bisexual men is leveling off, and perhaps even decreasing. In 1991, for example, 24,216 men were diagnosed with HIV/AIDS in the exposure category of men having sex with men; in 1992, there were 23,936 men diagnosed in the same category (Centers for Disease Control 1993b). This slight decline reflects a number of factors, including significant changes in sexual behavior among large com-

5

munities of gay and bisexual men, and increases in the quality of life for HIV-infected people, prior to the onset of AIDS, as a result of effective antiviral therapies.

Although the slight decline of HIV/AIDS within the gay and bisexual male population is a positive trend, there will continue to be a large number of new cases of HIV/AIDS for decades to come, and it remains to be seen whether the trend can be maintained over time. Experts are reinforcing the need for continued funding for HIV prevention efforts within the gay and bisexual male population, particularly for gay male youth, gay men of color, and men who have sex with men but who do not identify themselves as gay, and who therefore might not have access to prevention messages in the "mainstream" gay men's community (Freudenberg 1989).

The incidence of HIV/AIDS among heterosexual injection drug users, while still increasing slightly, may be leveling off. While 11,314 people were diagnosed with HIV/AIDS in the exposure category of injection drug users in 1991, and 11,425 were diagnosed in 1992, only one-quarter of the new cases involved women (Centers for Disease Control 1993b).

The incidence of HIV/AIDS among women with HIV-infected sexual partners, however, continues to rise, as does the incidence among babies born to HIV-infected mothers. These infection levels are occurring primarily in inner cities and among the poor in rural areas. While the annual number of cases among all people 20 years to 29 years old increased by 15.5 percent, the annual number of 20- to 29-year-old women with heterosexually acquired AIDS increased by 96.7 percent. This trend was greater among African American women than Caucasian or Hispanic women (Centers for Disease Control 1993b).

African American and Hispanic women compose a disproportionately large percentage of all HIV-infected women. As the incidence levels grow within these minority populations, the complexity of the overall social and health care problems facing HIV-infected people is increasing. As the National Research Council (1993) points out:

> A constant theme ... of the HIV/AIDS literature is the stigma, discrimination, and inequalities of the HIV/AIDS pandemic. At its outset, HIV disease settled among socially de-

valued groups, and as the pandemic has progressed, HIV/AIDS has increasingly been an affliction of people who have little economic, political, and social power.

As medical technology improves, some sources of HIV transmission should be entirely preventable. For example, transmission of HIV through blood transfusion is close to eradication as a result of autogenous transfusions and testing for HIV antibodies, which began in 1985.

Geographic Distribution

Distribution of both HIV/AIDS cases and HIV antibody prevalence varies substantially by geographic area (Centers for Disease Control 1987b). The incidence of disease is much higher in urban than in rural populations, although the incidence is rising in the rural South (Centers for Disease Control 1993b). The geographic distribution of HIV infection differs among specific groups with high-risk behavior (Centers for Disease Control 1987b). Data for persons with hemophilia indicate high levels of infection regardless of area.

Prevalence levels vary among homosexual and bisexual men, with the highest levels observed in California and the Northeast. HIV antibody prevalence among injection drug users varies widely: incidence is highest in Puerto Rico and the New York City area, moderately high elsewhere on the East Coast and in California, and generally below 5 percent in most other areas of the country (Centers for Disease Control 1987b).

Age

The number of reported AIDS cases in the United States varies according to age, reflecting the transmission patterns of the disease. The largest number of cases occurs in the 25- to 45-year-old group, representing the exposure categories of those who acquired HIV through unprotected sexual activity and, to a lesser extent, those who acquired HIV through injection drug use. Although the cases in these two exposure categories cluster in this age group, they extend from adolescence through old age. Another distinctly age-related group is that of infants who acquired HIV perinatally. In other exposure categories—such as recipients of transfusions—the cases are more evenly distributed across age groups.

HIV seroprevalence data also follow these age-related trends and give us more immediate information about the trends of the epidemic than can be gleaned from actual cases of AIDS, for which infection often occurred more than 10 years ago. However, HIV seroprevalence is only measured in discrete population groups, making generalization to the overall population impossible. The group that is perhaps the least studied is children below the age of 16 years. We know more about adolescents as they reach young adulthood: in 1989, the seroprevalence among Job Corps applicants 16 years to 21 years of age was 3.9/1,000, and among college students using health services at 13 campuses was 2/1,000 (Hein 1992).

Of great concern is the fact that these increases are concentrated in certain exposure categories. A cumulative total of 1,301 13- to 19-year-olds with AIDS had been reported to the CDC by the end of June 1993. Nearly one-quarter of these were young men who acquired HIV infection through homosexual contact. Of the other teens, 30 percent acquired HIV as a result of treatment for their hemophilia, 18 percent acquired HIV through heterosexual contact, 11 percent acquired HIV through injection drug use, 6 percent received HIV-infected blood transfusions, 3 percent were in the dual category of gay/bisexual men and injection drug users, and 7 percent had an undetermined source of HIV infection (Centers for Disease Control 1992).

The increasing incidence of HIV/AIDS among adolescents is causing the potential productive work force to decline in comparison with the elderly population — profoundly affecting the future of our society as we prepare to enter the 21st century. According to Hein (1992), AIDS is the ninth leading cause of death among children 1 year to 4 years of age, and the sixth in young people between the ages of 15 and 24. In the latter age group, AIDS deaths have increased 100-fold between 1981 and 1987. If current trends continue, AIDS could well be among the top five causes of death for young people ages 15 years to 24 years in the next few years.

Gender

As of January 1993, 88 percent of all reported cases of HIV/AIDS in the United States involved men (Centers for Disease Control 1993b). This statistic reflects the fact that 63 percent of these cases occurred among gay and bisexual men. Earlier in the pandemic, the percentage of HIV/AIDS cases among men was even higher, but it has gradually declined. The male-to-female ratio of reported HIV/AIDS cases in 1984 was 14:1, compared to 7:1 in 1991 (Mann, Tarantola, and Netter 1992).

On the other hand, the incidence of HIV/AIDS among women continues to rise. In 1991, 5,732 women were diagnosed with HIV/AIDS; that number had risen to 6,255 by 1992. This increase particularly reflects the growing number of women whose exposure category is heterosexual contact with HIV-infected men (Centers for Disease Control 1993b). In 1992, HIV/AIDS was the fifth leading cause of death among young women in the United States. HIV seropositivity is now nearly equal among men and women in several tested populations in the United States, including groups of armed service recruits, certain urban populations, Job Corps candidates, and armed service reservists.

Race and Ethnicity

The HIV/AIDS pandemic is having a disproportionate impact on African Americans and Hispanics as compared with Caucasians. Although African Americans constituted only 12 percent of the U.S. population as of December 1992, they accounted for 30 percent of all reported cases of HIV/AIDS, and for 54 percent of all reported pediatric cases of HIV/AIDS. Additionally, although Hispanics constituted only 9 percent of the U.S. population, they accounted for 17 percent of all reported cases of HIV/AIDS, and for 24 percent of all reported pediatric cases.

During the same time period, Caucasians made up over 75 percent of the U.S. population, yet accounted for only 52 percent of all reported cases of HIV/AIDS, and for 20 percent of all reported pediatric cases (Centers for Disease Control 1993b; National Commission on AIDS 1992). As early as 1988, HIV/AIDS was the leading cause of death among African American women aged 15 years to 44 years in the states of New York and New Jersey (Centers for Disease Control 1991c).

Native Americans and Asian Americans/Pacific Islanders are under-represented among HIV/AIDS cases in proportion to their numbers in the total population. As of September 1992, Asian Americans/Pacific Islanders—who constitute 3 percent of the U.S. population—accounted for only 0.6 percent of the HIV/AIDS cases reported to the CDC. Similarly, Native Americans, who constitute 0.8 percent of the U.S. population, accounted for only 0.17 percent of the reported HIV/AIDS cases.

There is cause for concern, however, that these communities are still in the early stages of a growing HIV pandemic. According to the National Commission on AIDS (1992):

> Because of their relative insularity, which magnifies the effect of infectious diseases once they take hold, the course of the pandemic in these communities could come to resemble that of the African American and Hispanic/Latino populations if effective prevention interventions are not brought to bear.

In fact, there is evidence that this is already occurring among Native Americans. From 1989 to 1990, the number of HIV/AIDS cases reported among Native Americans increased faster than cases among any other ethnic or racial group. HIV/AIDS cases among Native Americans rose 23 percent, compared with 13 percent for Hispanics/Latinos, 12 percent for African Americans, and 2.5 percent for Caucasians. Additionally, studies of applicants for military service from 1985 to 1990 indicate that Native American male recruits had a seropositivity rate twice that of Caucasian male recruits (National Commission on AIDS 1992).

There is no evidence that race is a biological risk factor for HIV infection. The heavy impact on some ethnic and racial minorities can be attributed to the same factors that cause high infant and maternal mortality rates and high rates of sexually transmitted diseases among some groups—lack of access to education, employment, decent housing, and adequate health care. Racism perpetuates urban and rural ghettos, which become impoverished communities where opportunities are scarce, drug use is rampant, and disease spreads quickly.

Tuberculosis

Tuberculosis (TB) is a chronic pulmonary and extrapulmonary infectious disease caused by *Mycobacterium tuberculosis* (MTB). In many U.S. cities, there has been a dramatic rise in the incidence of active tuberculosis, which is found in people who are homeless, drug addicted, and/or immigrants from countries where TB is endemic. Specifically, the incidence of TB has increased among people with HIV infection, both because of reactivation of old TB infection when the immune system becomes compromised and because of new TB infection when the person with HIV/AIDS is exposed to a person with active TB disease. Extrapulmonary dissemination of tuberculosis can involve lymph nodes, bone marrow, the central nervous system, and the genitourinary tract.

Although people with HIV infection are no more likely than other people to acquire TB infection when exposed to it, they *are* more likely to develop full-blown TB disease once they become infected, and to have a fulminant course of the disease. It is recommended that all people with HIV infection be screened for TB with an anergy panel and, if purified-protein-derivative (PPD)-positive, be considered for TB prophylaxis. Additionally, people found to be PPD-positive, especially younger individuals, should be counseled regarding possible HIV testing.

Even with TB infection, an HIV-positive person may not react to the PPD test, and chest X-rays may not show characteristic changes in persons with severely depressed immune systems. Therefore, clinical symptoms, such as cough, fever, weight loss, night sweats, and fatigue, become important indicators that an immune-depressed person might have TB. To check for false negative PPD results, anergy testing should be done routinely on HIV-positive persons.

The danger of nurses acquiring TB from patients has increased in recent years. As the public health system has experienced funding cutbacks, there has been insufficient follow-up of TB patients to assure compliance with drug treatment. This has resulted in the development of *multidrug-resistant* strains of TB (MDR-TB). Immuno-compromised health care workers have died after acquiring MDR-TB from people with HIV/AIDS (Centers for Disease Control 1991d).

Any discussion of mycobacterial infection in a person with HIV infection would be incomplete without reference to *Mycobacterium avium complex* (MAC), which is not transmitted person-to-person as in MTB. MAC causes disseminated disease in up to 40 percent of patients with advanced HIV disease in the United States. Effective prevention of and therapy for MAC have the potential to contribute to an improved quality of life and duration of survival for HIV-infected persons (Centers for Disease Control 1991d).

International Epidemiology

As of December 1992, a total of 611,589 cases of HIV/AIDS were reported to the World Health Organization (WHO) from 168 countries throughout the world. However, significant under-reporting in many areas of the world means that this number is actually low. In fact, WHO estimates that the total number of HIV/AIDS cases in the world at the end of 1992 was 2.5 million, and that an additional 13 million people were infected with the HIV/AIDS virus. This is an increase 120 times over the 100,000 people estimated as infected in 1980 (Mann, Tarantola, and Netter 1992).

On a population basis, the most heavily affected areas of the world are sub-Saharan Africa, the Caribbean, North America, and Latin America. The Global HIV/AIDS Policy Coalition (GAPC) at Harvard University estimates that 40 percent of all HIV-infected adults worldwide are women. Of the estimated worldwide total of 1.1 million children infected with HIV, 90 percent live in sub-Saharan Africa, 4 percent in Latin America, 2 percent in Southeast Asia, and 1.5 percent in North America (Mann, Tarantola, and Netter 1992).

The primary mode of transmission differs significantly in various parts of the world. According to GAPC estimates, 56 percent of infected North American adults acquired HIV through male-to-male sex, and 27 percent through injection drug use. In sub-Saharan

Africa, on the other hand, 93 percent of HIV infection was acquired through heterosexual sex (Mann 1992).

By 1995, it is estimated that there will be nearly 17.5 million adults worldwide infected with HIV, and more than 2.2 million HIV-infected children. In a study of 10 countries in Central and East Africa, the United Nations Children's Fund (UNICEF) projects that by 1999, HIV/AIDS will have orphaned nearly 11 percent of the population of those countries, and will account for an increase of as much as 43 percent in the deaths of children under five years old (Mann, Tarantola, and Netter 1992).

2

Ethical Perspectives

The Care of Persons with HIV/AIDS

Ethical considerations related to the care of persons with HIV/AIDS have evolved with the pandemic. In the early 1980s, nurses were concerned primarily with two issues: 1) whether nurses were responsible for giving nursing care to HIV-infected individuals, and 2) the protection of patient confidentiality. Today's pressing questions cover some prior concerns, but also include many new ethical dilemmas, including:

- mandatory HIV testing for patients and health care workers,
- specialized or integrated HIV/AIDS delivery systems,
- drug testing for treatment modalities,
- concentrating goods and resources on patients with early- or late-stage disease,
- reporting HIV-positive persons to public health/government agencies and/or employers, and
- confidentiality/disclosure limits and responsibilities.

HIV/AIDS has made the possible transmission of a fatal disease a reality for the first time in most American nurses' careers. The ethical questions to be considered are very real, challenging, and often confusing for nurses. The *Code for Nurses with Interpretive Statements* makes explicit the values and ethical precepts of the profession, and provides guidance for conduct and relationships in carrying out nursing actions (American Nurses Association 1985).

Within the framework of the *Code for Nurses*, nurses can make ethical decisions and discharge their professional responsibilities. The *Code for Nurses* states that the "nurse provides services with respect for human dignity and the uniqueness of the person, unrestricted by consideration of social or economic status, personal attributes, or the nature of health problems" (American Nurses Association 1985). There is a profound commitment both by the profession and the individual practitioner to these fundamental principles of respect for persons and the right to self-determination.

Nurses have a responsibility to understand the complex ethical dimensions of practice, to seek solutions, and to work within their individual settings for the provision of nonjudgmental, compassionate, and competent care to people with HIV infection. The nurse will need to reexamine his or her value system continually and challenge preconceptions in order to respond appropriately to the needs of the person with HIV/AIDS. In the opinion of Kristine Gebbie, National AIDS Policy Coordinator, "Nurses represent a kind of creativity that combines the best of what we already know and the best of what can be brought out to provide care, education, and research" (Gebbie 1990).

The question of mandatory versus voluntary testing of patients and health care workers and the fear of possible discrimination has raised ethical concerns and become a major political and social issue. Additional ethical concerns include:

- What is the most efficient and effective use of limited resources?
- Should care be delivered in centralized or integrated HIV/AIDS inpatient units?
- What is the nurse's responsibility in experimental treatment protocols and alternative treatment models?
- Should HIV-positive persons be reported by name?
- What are the parameters for disclosure of HIV/AIDS status to individuals who are at risk for disease transmission?

Controversy and confusion surround these issues, and it is apparent that there are no easy answers. Nurses will encounter inaccuracies, fears, and myths associated with HIV/AIDS, and will need to examine their professional and ethical responses carefully.

Nurses must work with other health care professionals to provide assistance and education to policy makers, legislators, and civic leaders in promoting community and national efforts to meet the health needs of people with HIV/AIDS. With the numerous ethical questions to be addressed in HIV/AIDS care, and with new ones arising each day, professional associations, state and local policy makers, advocacy groups, health care facilities, and individual caregivers all face complex and intense decisions.

June Osborn, the 1989-1993 Chairperson of the National Commission on AIDS, summed up these difficulties by stating that, "HIV/AIDS, more than any other disease, has crystallized for Americans all that is complex, good, and bad in our health care and society" (National Commission on AIDS 1992). The ethical issues of HIV/AIDS certainly crystallize the many challenges for nurses in providing care to HIV-infected persons.

Health Care Workers

The fundamental ethical principles expressed in the *Code for Nurses* (American Nurses Association 1985) provide direction and guidance to assist the nurse in making appropriate decisions in the workplace. Since the beginning of the pandemic, nurses have provided care and support for people with HIV/AIDS in clinics, hospitals, homes, schools, nursing homes, and shelters. Nurses recognize a primary commitment to the health, welfare, and safety of individuals with HIV/AIDS.

While the obligation to care for all people is integral to the practice of nursing, it is important to recognize that some nurses remain fearful of carrying out this responsibility with regard to HIV/AIDS patients. Scientific evidence has demonstrated that the risk of transmission of HIV/AIDS is exceedingly low when proper precautions are employed (Centers for Disease Control 1989). Nurses can safeguard patients and themselves through adherence to universal precautions and infectious disease guidelines. Nurses can further this safeguarding obligation by educating other health care providers, monitoring practice, and participating in the development of institutional policies and procedures.

The presence of an HIV-positive health care provider in the workplace creates new ethical concerns. Nurses who know that they are HIV-infected should voluntarily avoid exposure-prone invasive procedures that have been scientifically linked to HIV or other blood-borne infection transmission. Self-restriction of practice must be decided on a case-by-case basis through consultation with the personal care provider and in keeping with guidelines from the CDC and state professional boards [see Appendix A]. Confidentiality of information about HIV-infected nurses must be maintained. Except in situations where a patient clearly has been exposed to an HIV-infected nurse's blood, the nurse should not be required to disclose his or her infection status.

3

Social Context

The Client

The client is any individual, family, or community with the potential for exposure to HIV, or experiencing symptoms related to HIV infection. Clients with HIV infection come from all segments of society. Currently, gay/bisexual men, African Americans, and Hispanics represent a disproportionate percentage of HIV-infected people, compared with the total population.

As the first identified HIV/AIDS risk group, gay/bisexual men encountered a strong resurgence in homophobia. Their strong community and political organization, effective advocacy, and organized leadership were crucial in alerting other members of society to the dangers and complex social issues accompanying HIV/AIDS, and to the need for behavior changes to decrease risk.

Increasing numbers of children, adolescents, and women are being diagnosed with HIV infection. Primarily from minority groups, they often must also deal with problems related to poverty, substance abuse, and inadequate health care. Many children come from families where one or both parents and/or siblings may be infected. Many other individuals are without families or have been abandoned. A group starting to receive more recognition is older adults, an increasing percentage of whom are infected with HIV (Moss and Miles 1987).

The Family

Within the context of HIV/AIDS care, it is important to recognize the meaning of "family" in its broadest sense—the group of people who form the innermost support network for the person with HIV infection. The family of a person with HIV infection may be traditional (e.g., a husband and wife), nontraditional (e.g., a gay man and his lover), or nonexistent (e.g., an estranged homeless person). The family members often have a mixture of biological, legal, and emotional ties with the HIV-infected person. For example, one person with HIV infection may consider her family to be her boyfriend, her children, and her mother. Another person with HIV infection may consider his family to be his sister, his best friend, and a volunteer who visits him from a local HIV/AIDS service organization.

The nurse should consider the entire family as being affected by the HIV/AIDS infection, and should include them in treatment plans if the person with HIV agrees. Legal considerations, such as the federal Patient Self-Determination Act, and institutional policies, such as visiting rights, should be implemented in relation to the HIV-infected person's designated family.

The family may include more than one person who is HIV-infected. If a person who is infected is a caregiver for children or for another sick person in the family, problems may arise in meeting the possibly conflicting needs of these various dependent people. For instance, children who are HIV-infected may require more attention than healthy children.

The family often provides the ongoing, day-to-day, and crisis support needed by a person with HIV infection. Families, health care providers, and support agencies must recognize that they also need support to maintain increasingly demanding caregiving functions.

The Caregiver

Caregivers for people with HIV infection include both paid health care providers, such as nurses and home health attendants, and personal caregivers, such as family members, friends, and volunteers. For all of these people, the intense needs of a person who suffers from HIV/AIDS can be overwhelming, particularly in the long-run. Reduction in the ability to cope (i.e., *burnout*) is a constant danger unless actions are taken to prevent it. Each caregiver's physical and emotional limits must be acknowledged and respected. Respite should be provided for day-to-day caregivers in the home or hospice setting, and support groups should be available for both health care providers and personal caregivers.

The School

The number of HIV-infected babies being born in the United States is increasing, and more and more of these children are living longer. In a retrospective study of HIV-infected babies, half of them lived to be more than five years old (Krasinski, Borkowsky, and Holzman 1989). Every HIV-infected child requires socialization with other children for optimum growth and development, whether or not the HIV infection slows down normal developmental milestones. Day care facilities should provide socialization opportunities for the child and respite for the parent. Primary and secondary schools should support these opportunities for the older child or adolescent along with his or her education.

Society has initially resisted the participation of HIV-infected children in day care and school settings because of fears that other children would become infected. There have been countless worldwide examples of parent groups organizing angry school boycotts when it became known that a child with HIV infection was going to enroll in their local school system. Vigorous education of the community is usually necessary to overcome the fear of children with HIV/AIDS.

The Centers for Disease Control and Prevention have provided guidelines on the education of children infected with HIV. These guidelines state that there is no apparent risk of HIV transmission among school-age children who have no neurological or behavioral impairments, and that HIV-infected children should be allowed to attend school. However, a more restricted environment is recommended by the CDC for preschool-age children and neurologically handicapped children. A team composed of the child's parents, physician, school nurse, and public health and school personnel should consider each situation individually. The confidentiality and privacy of the child should be maintained, with the minimum number of school personnel being made aware of the child's condition (Centers for Disease Control 1985).

The Community

There has been a tremendous stigma attached to HIV infection in communities throughout the world, based on the fear of contagion and on moral judgment of the sexual and drug-using behaviors often associated with transmission. However, there also has been a social response of compassion and caring within the same communities. In fact, many have been strengthened through people coming together to cope with the impact of the disease on individuals and community. Community-based organizations have been formed, both formally and informally, to educate those at risk for HIV infection and to care for those who already are infected. Many religious organizations have focused efforts on individuals and families suffering from the effects of HIV.

The HIV/AIDS pandemic has been described as dynamic and complex (Mann, Tarantola, and Netter 1992). The related psychosocial challenges will be great, both in communities experiencing the pandemic for the first time and in communities in which the initial shock is over and ongoing devastation is occurring.

As HIV affects new groups of people, each new community responds in a similar manner. The first response usually is denial, whereby individuals identify the risk behaviors as belonging to other people to assure themselves that they are not vulnerable to infection. For prevention efforts to be effective, education must confront this denial and assist individuals in recognizing that they *are* at risk. This education is most effective when implemented by members of the community.

The first individuals to become infected with HIV generally experience stigmatization and isolation because of the community's denial and fear. As more people become ill, and more individuals therefore have personal experience with the suffering caused by HIV/

AIDS, the community is able to acknowledge that the pandemic is indeed a reality.

More and more people are required to become caregivers for their loved ones; more and more community resources are directed to meet the health care, financial, and psychosocial needs of affected people; and the community as a whole begins to experience the terrible and overwhelming impact of the pandemic. The communities of gay men in major cities in the United States have reached this stage, and burnout among professional and personal caregivers is a critical issue. The sense of hopelessness and despair must be addressed on both individual and community levels to enable the community to continue coping with and responding to the pandemic.

4

Prevention of HIV Infection

The Role of the Nurse in HIV Prevention

As both a professional and a member of the community, the nurse has the authority and the obligation to influence the community's response to the HIV pandemic. The nurse can assist in the development of prevention and treatment programs that meet the needs of those at risk and those infected with HIV within a given community.

The primary AIDS-related public health goal is to prevent HIV transmission. As already described, HIV is primarily transmitted through unsafe sexual practices with an infected partner or through the sharing of needles. Because there currently is no vaccine for HIV infection, education to change risk behavior is the only method available to help prevent its transmission.

Nurses practice in many diverse settings—schools, clinics, private health care offices, shelters, long-term care institutions, senior centers, neighborhood health centers, health maintenance organizations (HMOs), hospitals, homes, and occupational settings. This variety of settings provides nurses with the unique opportunity to educate individuals about risk behaviors and methods to prevent HIV infection at multiple points of contact with the health and social service systems.

Practicing in different settings also gives professional nurses the opportunity to educate other health care workers—as well as colleagues in related occupations, such as police and fire department personnel—about HIV Workplace education should include not only basic information about HIV transmission and prevention, but also information about the problems and needs of persons with HIV/AIDS, along with facts about the transmission and prevention of *all* bloodborne diseases in the workplace.

Risk Assessment

To provide prevention education to high-risk individuals, nurses must be able to assess levels of risk for HIV infection correctly. Certain individuals, such as homosexual men and injection drug users, may identify themselves as being at high risk for acquiring HIV. But many other people either do not acknowledge that their behavior puts them at risk for HIV (e.g., men who occasionally have sex with men), or are not aware that their behavior is putting them at risk in the first place (e.g., women who do not know their sexual partners inject drugs and/or have other partners, and who only discover HIV infection when their child is diagnosed). To reach these people, information and education about HIV transmission and prevention must continue to be targeted to *all* members of the community, and risk assessments must be completed on *all* persons encountered by nurses in their practice settings.

Nurses must develop comfort and expertise in discussing sexual behaviors and alcohol or drug use (including injection drug use) with their clients. Educational programs should provide nurses not only with information, but also with opportunities to explore their personal attitudes and to practice interviewing clients through role-playing.

Many people who engage in risky behaviors need assistance to admit that they are at risk for HIV. For these people, going through a risk assessment with a supportive health care professional can be an instructive experience and can provide the necessary motivation to seek out resources for behavior change, including counseling and HIV testing.

Personal Risk Avoidance/Risk Reduction

Educating individuals on how to avoid or reduce the risk of HIV is crucial once their risk of exposure to HIV has been assessed. There are strong indications that carefully targeted educational programs and individual health counseling directed at changing high-risk behaviors have been effective in combating the transmission of HIV (Becker and Joseph 1988). Educational efforts directed toward changing sexual and/or drug use behavior continue to be crucial, and should be culturally specific and developmentally appropriate (Kalichman et al. 1993). To assure effectiveness, educational programs must be regularly evaluated, and appropriate changes in the program or intervention must be made based on the evaluation (Coyle, Boruch, and Turner 1991; Moulton et al. 1989).

Not only should women of childbearing age be counseled about changing risky behavior to prevent HIV transmission, they also should be informed about the potential for perinatal transmission of HIV (estimated at 30 percent) if they become HIV-positive. The seropositive woman should be informed and counseled about the risk of perinatal transmission and offered information about contraception.

Counseling and health education concepts and strategies have been applied in a variety of programs to assist at-risk individuals in changing their behaviors. Many strategies—such as skills development, values clarification, self-esteem building, and assertiveness training—have been used effectively with people with HIV/AIDS, both in individual and group settings. Specific activities such as role-playing and small group discussion have been found useful in implementing these strategies.

One-to-one and group counseling lie at the heart of many HIV prevention interventions, whether this occurs through a telephone hot line or a walk-in service center. Training community members to become peer counselors has been shown to be very effective within local communities. Peer counseling can occur in structured sessions at an agency or through informal contact in the community. Many HIV prevention programs hire street outreach workers who engage in peer counseling with individuals at risk for HIV infection, such as injection drug users or commercial sex workers.

Behavior change counseling involves developing relationships with individuals and working with them to assess their personal level of risk for HIV infection, to identify the problems resulting in risky behavior, to identify potential solutions to those problems, and to select and apply solutions that are individually appropriate.

Social influence is increasingly being seen as an important component of effecting behavior change among at-risk individuals, particularly adolescents (Fisher and Misovich 1990). An HIV education intervention that is used successfully in many communities involves training peer educators, who then invite a group of their friends to a house party where HIV education and discussion about personal risk are combined in a warm, safe environment. The Stop AIDS Project in San Francisco, developed within the gay men's community, is an example of this model. The use of community leaders to initiate change in behavioral norms is another social influence strategy that has been proven effective (Kelly et al. 1991).

Several programs that focus on specific populations with the potential for participating in risk behaviors have successfully addressed the cultural and age-specific needs of different individuals. The Pilsen Catholic Youth Center in Chicago's Latino community, for instance, is training young people aged 16 years to 21 years to be AIDS peer educators in their own neighborhoods. In another example, the Bayview-Hunter's Point Foundation and the San Francisco Health Department used a rap contest to reach potentially at-risk teenagers, and to enable them to reach each other. A key strategy for engaging young people is to use their own energy and enthusiasm to create momentum for HIV/AIDS education (Freudenberg 1989).

Programs that target ethnic minority populations use positive elements of their own cultures for HIV education. For example, "Blacks Educating Blacks about Sexual Health Issues" (BEBASHI) in Philadelphia, which works in the African American community, uses examples of families and children in their AIDS education programs (Freudenberg 1989). Other minority-focused HIV prevention agencies work within existing community organizations, such as churches and tenant groups, and approach elected officials, ministers, and health professionals to deliver AIDS education messages.

Many HIV education programs have been implemented, but none can provide conclusive evidence that the interventions actually work because impact evaluation has not been done. Evaluation of these programs and publication of the findings is necessary to provide data that will enable the health care community to develop and refine programs to facilitate behavior changes in persons engaging in high-risk behaviors (Coyle, Boruch, and Turner 1991).

HIV *Counseling and Testing*

When HIV testing is a component of the practice setting, pre- and post-test counseling are essential aspects of the process. Counseling reduces the person's anxiety, elicits a personal risk assessment, provides relevant information about the test and about HIV prevention, and assures that the person receives appropriate support and referrals depending on whether the test is positive or negative (Kraut 1987). HIV counseling and testing opportunities are offered within health care practices, and also within health department and community-based clinics. In most states, anonymous counseling and testing (where a person does not divulge his or her name and is provided services anonymously) is offered in certain settings.

Protecting the confidentiality of HIV test results has been acomplished differently in various states and health institutions. However, these test results often are considered to require more stringent protections than other aspects of the health care record because of the potential for discrimination in housing, employment, health insurance, and health care itself as a result of disclosure of positive HIV status. Numerous situations have been documented in which individuals have been evicted from housing, have lost jobs and health insurance, and/or have not received appropriate health care as a result of the disclosure of a positive HIV test (Feldblum 1992).

In states where an individual's HIV test result is kept separate from his or her medical record and not made known to health care providers other than the physician who ordered the test, confidentiality continues to be a contentious issue among health care providers. It is generally felt that the primary care nurse, in addition to the physician, needs to know the HIV status of the person with HIV infection in order to provide appropriate, comprehensive, and humane care. Also, the nurse providing direct care may need to know the person's status to provide comprehensive nursing care, including meeting the psychosocial and emotional needs of the person with HIV/AIDS. In this context, awareness of the significance of confidentiality and of the repercussions of disclosure is vital.

In addition to confidentiality, another important HIV testing issue involves voluntary versus mandatory testing. The ANA House of Delegates supports the availability of voluntary, anonymous testing with informed consent and appropriate counseling (see Appendix A). Individuals seeking services at drug rehabilitation clinics, sexually transmitted disease clinics, prenatal clinics, TB clinics, or family planning clinics should have access to confidential testing and counseling about health practices. Confidentiality of test results must be maintained to prevent discrimination.

Regardless of whether individuals are found to be seronegative or seropositive, targeted health education and individual counseling programs—addressing positive health practices and the avoidance of high-risk behaviors—must be provided by qualified health professionals. The decision to be tested must be made by choice rather than coercion, and must be made by individuals who have been appropriately counseled (see Appendix A).

Occupational Risk Avoidance/ Risk Reduction

The Occupational Safety and Health Administration's (OSHA) bloodborne pathogen standard requires employers to provide an exposure control plan, engineering controls, personal protective equipment, hepatitis B immunization, hazard communication, exposure follow-up and treatment, and education and training regarding occupational risk and risk education. This standard generally prohibits two-handed recapping of syringes, and strongly encourages the increased use of safety devices such as safety syringes and needleless IV systems. Employers are required to evaluate current technology in relation to exposure-related events.

Current studies on HIV infection control document the need for behavior changes among health care workers in order to improve the manner in which infection control and safety techniques are practiced (Gerberding 1986; Gerberding et al. 1987; Henderson et al. 1986). Ongoing educational programs specifically targeted to health care workers should facilitate the essential behavior changes. These educational programs must emphasize the need to use infection control precautions with *all* exposures to blood and body fluids (Centers for Disease Control 1987c), although workplace safety precautions also require the development and availability of equipment to reduce the risk of exposure to bloodborne pathogens in the first place (see Appendix A).

The CDC's recommendations for universal precautions to prevent the transmission of HIV infection must be implemented during care of all persons (Centers for Disease Control 1987c). Any person can be infected with HIV and have no symptoms; therefore, blood and body fluid precautions are appropriate with *all* persons to protect health care workers and other patients from exposure to HIV/AIDS and other bloodborne infectious organisms. Although the risk of HIV transmission to health care workers is extremely small, nurses must be vigilant regarding the implementation of CDC guidelines (Centers for Disease Control 1987c) (see Appendix D). The implementation of these recommendations is not a deterrent to the provision of quality care.

Nurses also can provide leadership in educating their families, peers, students, other health care providers, and the nursing profession at large about preventive strategies. The family members and students of nurses have many of the same misconceptions about HIV/AIDS as the general community, and often experience fear about their family member or teacher providing nursing care in an environment perceived to be unsafe. Education programs directed toward family members and friends may alleviate common fears and facilitate support for individuals engaged in or considering nursing as a career.

The Health Promotion and Management of Persons with HIV/AIDS

Care along the HIV/AIDS Spectrum

Nursing involves practices that are nurturing, generative, preventive, and protective in nature. Nursing care provided to HIV-infected individuals must be in full accordance with the *Standards of Clinical Nursing Practice* (American Nurses Association 1991). The HIV pandemic is stimulating the development of nontraditional models of care. In addition, scientific developments are occurring rapidly, creating a demand for nurses willing to develop expertise in the care of persons with HIV infection.

HIV/AIDS is actually a spectrum of conditions—an HIV-infected individual usually progresses systematically from completely asymptomatic HIV infection to full-blown AIDS. There are individuals who live many years after an HIV-positive diagnosis, and even after an AIDS diagnosis. All people living with HIV/AIDS need to be seen as individuals rather than statistical probabilities. The nurse must be able to assess the individual's psychological and physical status, as well as his or her needs at each stage of the disease process. For a person who is asymptomatic, care may involve the provision of information on health maintenance, and referrals for emotional and social support. For a person on the other end of the spectrum, a multidisciplinary team involving multiple agencies may need to work together to meet his or her extensive care needs.

Treatment

As the immune dysfunction associated with HIV disease becomes better understood, interventions in the early stages of HIV disease—such as prophylaxis for particular opportunistic infections and antiviral therapies—are becoming part of standard clinical practice. Many people with HIV infection want access to clinical drug trials to gain access to new, potentially effective therapies. The nurse should know how to assist the person with HIV/AIDS in obtaining this access, and should take into consideration the fact that many other people with HIV/AIDS may be enrolled in clinical trials.

Intensive medical research efforts are being directed toward vaccine development, antiviral therapies, and the prevention and treatment of opportunistic diseases. The nurse is challenged to remain up-to-date on rapidly changing protocols for the standard drugs used to treat HIV-related diseases, as well as on newly approved drugs and drugs still under investigation.

In addition to the experimental therapies being tested, many people with HIV infection use nonmedically prescribed therapies (often referred to as "alternative" or "complementary" therapies), including nutritional regimens, acupuncture, herbs and vitamins, and meditation. An important part of a nursing history is to obtain information about what therapies a person with HIV/AIDS is pursuing. Although the nursing scope of practice does not mandate training in alternative therapies, the nurse needs to be familiar with what alternative or complementary therapies are offered in the community to help the client assess the pros and cons of these other therapies in a nonjudgmental, supportive manner.

Psychological Support

People with HIV/AIDS face many issues that are emotionally challenging, including the stigma associated with HIV, the fear of abandonment, multiple losses over time, and the fact that AIDS is life-threatening. Assisting the person with HIV/AIDS to cope with these issues and with the disease itself is an integral aspect of the nursing process. Nurses have addressed these issues with people with HIV/

AIDS throughout the pandemic in a wide range of health care and community-based settings.

Nurses in all roles attend to psychological needs and provide referral and direct interventions to meet those needs. In attending to the whole person, the nurse should be skilled in the assessment of psychological needs, the planning and implementation of interventions to meet those needs, and the evaluation of the effectiveness of interventions.

The psychological assessment of the person with HIV/AIDS requires sensitivity to the impact of HIV on the individual, as well as the role that the individual's cultural background and lifestyle play in this impact. The nurse must initially assess the emotional condition and internal resources of both the individual and the family, not only in terms of long-term planning, but also in terms of potential crisis intervention.

Suicidal ideation may occur with the person who has just learned of his or her HIV status. Depression is found among people experiencing the loss of body functions and, concomitantly, the loss of roles within the family and within society. Anxiety and hopelessness are among the conditions that can lead to dysfunctional coping responses to the disease process. In each individual situation, it is important to assess whether responses such as denial or anger are healthy coping methods or are counterproductive to the well-being of the person with HIV/AIDS. In addition, the nurse must be able to differentiate between psychological symptoms and HIV-related organic processes, such as dementia.

Nursing interventions based on the psychosocial assessment should be person-centered. They should be developed in conjunction with the person with HIV/AIDS and the family, if possible. The overriding sense of helplessness related to HIV disease can only be addressed by providing as much control as possible to the person with HIV/AIDS. Most likely, interventions will include referral to resources in the community, particularly HIV-related resources. In addition, interventions may include intense involvement with the person with HIV/AIDS over time, possibly along with an interdisciplinary team of providers. HIV is a complex disease with multiple psychosocial implications, and a number of disciplines may be necessary to meet all of the needs of the person with HIV/AIDS.

Persons with HIV/AIDS face specific issues related to their sexual orientation, gender, and racial/ethnic backgrounds—all of which constitute part of each person's psychosocial picture. These issues must be clarified and acknowledged in assisting the person with HIV/AIDS to cope with the disease. For example, a man who has sex with men may or may not identify himself as being gay, and thus may or may not have access to the system of support provided within the gay community for persons with HIV/AIDS. A woman may feel compelled to hide the fact that she is HIV-infected because the assumption in her community may be that a woman who gets AIDS must be a prostitute. An African American with AIDS may not feel comfortable at local AIDS support groups composed only of Caucasians.

The psychological issues of HIV disease require nurses at each point of patient contact with the health care system to be intensely involved with the person with HIV/AIDS and the family. To provide the necessary ongoing psychological support to individuals with HIV/AIDS, nurses also require support. Facilities and agencies that have high HIV-related caseloads often provide support groups for staff, sometimes facilitated by a mental health provider (for example, a psychiatric nurse, psychologist, or social worker). Other support measures that have been helpful to providers working with HIV/AIDS patients include:

- encouraging staff to attend stress reduction workshops or HIV-related courses;
- providing after-hours social events; and/or
- encouraging staff to attend memorial services and funerals for individuals with HIV/AIDS with whom they have worked closely.

Substance Abuse Treatment

An issue of particular importance in relation to HIV is that of substance abuse. As of June 1993, 24 percent of the people reported to have AIDS in this country contracted HIV as a direct result of injection drug use (Centers for Disease Control 1993a). Many more either had a substance abuse problem prior to contracting HIV or began abusing drugs or alcohol after their diagnosis as a means of coping.

The patterns of behavior involved in abusing either drugs or alcohol often prevent the HIV-positive person from being able to cooperate with necessary treatment regimens and other aspects of a healthy lifestyle, and also prevent him or her from being able to avoid infecting others. In short, substance abuse often must be treated first in order to be able to treat the underlying HIV disease effectively. Nurses must be skilled in dealing with problems of addiction, and therefore able to work with appropriate community resources to provide nursing care to addicted people with HIV/AIDS.

Coordination of Care/Case Management

The medical and psychosocial needs of people with HIV/AIDS are complex and require a wide range of services. Early on in the epidemic, community-based organizations that provided support to persons with AIDS recognized that coordination of a multitude of services was needed. They began working closely with health care and social service institutions in new and innovative ways. The experience of the San Francisco community suggests a model of care for those with a complex disease that requires both hospitalization and home care—namely, the provision of community-based services with government money and support, and the use of both professional and volunteer staff (Jenna et al. 1988).

Nurses have always played a vital role in the development of community-based services. The development and maintenance of AIDS resource directories, assurance of the confidentiality of client records, education of personnel, and identification of funding resources are only a few of the critical areas needing input from nurses. Because of their understanding of the needs of persons with HIV/AIDS, nurses must be involved in the planning, development, and implementation of community resources and services.

In 1986, in response to the need for community services to be coordinated with established health and social services, and based on the successful community care model that was evolving in San Francisco, the Robert Wood Johnson Foundation funded demonstration projects to develop systems of coordinated care in 11 communities around the country.

In 1987, the Health Resources Services Administration (HRSA) followed suit and funded projects in several other communities. The result was a number of case-management models, ranging from a health-system-based, medically oriented approach, to a community-based, social services advocacy approach. In communities with extensive community-based resources, such as San Francisco, it was found that people with AIDS were discharged earlier from acute-care facilities than were patients with the same diagnosis seen in other communities, suggesting that coordination of care and the development of community-based services is cost-effective (Jenna 1987).

In 1990, the coordination of community services and the case-management approach to care were extended beyond these demonstration projects through the Ryan White Comprehensive AIDS Resources Emergency (CARE) Act. Case management was funded as a primary service, and coordination was facilitated by the implementation of planning councils and consortia under Titles I and II (Jonsen and Stryker 1993). In addition, pediatric demonstration projects were funded to coordinate care through case-management services at large hospitals such as the University of Miami-Jackson Memorial Hospital in Miami and Harlem Hospital in New York City (Jonsen and Stryker 1993).

Nurses play an important role in planning and implementing CARE-funded HIV/AIDS services throughout the country. Nurses providing care to persons with HIV infection within any health care setting should identify the services and resources available to their patients through the CARE Act. Care providers also should consider volunteering to participate on commissions or an HIV planning council as a member or resource person.

Case management for persons with HIV/AIDS is an activity that can utilize a wide range of nursing skills, including "client assessment and monitoring, coordination of the case management team, participation in interdisciplinary team meetings, health teaching of patients and caregivers, and preparing patients and families for managing potential deterioration" (Wright et al. 1993).

The need for interdisciplinary and interagency collaboration requires cooperation among multiple disciplines in a variety of settings. Colleagues from nursing, medicine, social work, psychology, religion, education, public health, and other disciplines all have a role to play in the delivery of care. Settings in which care is provided include homes, hospitals, clinics, mental health facilities, religious institutions, schools, prisons, long-term care facilities, hospices, and day care centers.

Coordination of care requires knowledge about the culturally-specific needs of the person with HIV/AIDS, and about existing programs available within the community. In the care and coordination of services for people with actual or potential HIV infection, the nurse utilizes knowledge acquired from an understanding of pathophysiology and psychosocial and cultural data, as well as from skills refined through providing direct patient care. The nurse utilizes his or her interpersonal skills in developing multidisciplinary approaches to meet the needs of persons with AIDS. Networking with community-based providers, public health agencies, schools, home health agencies, hospice programs, social service agencies, specialized AIDS services, and local legislators and officials provides numerous resources and opportunities to meet the needs of persons with HIV/AIDS, and to facilitate the effectiveness of prevention programs.

Advocacy for Persons with HIV/AIDS

Advocacy is an important component of the nurse's role in addressing the multiple and complex issues of prevention and care. Advocacy is necessary for the prevention of illness and for health promotion—both major nursing goals. Nurses practice in diverse settings that provide unique opportunities to 1) determine the needs of people at risk for HIV infection, 2) assess the quality and quantity of available resources, 3) determine the deficits in essential programs, and 4) advocate for initiation, expansion, or remediation of services.

People who have just discovered that they are seropositive should receive follow-up regarding health maintenance, as well as counseling related to the impact of the test result. The support of friends and family has been shown to benefit individuals coping with life-threatening illnesses. The nurse can assist in mobilizing these personal support systems.

In addition, nurses should become involved in advocating for the development of community support systems. There has been a notable lack of resources and services available for individuals from minority groups who are at risk or infected with HIV. There are many young people at risk for becoming infected as a result of their experimentation with unprotected sexual activity and/or injection drug use. There also are many chronically mentally ill and homeless people who may be impaired in their decision-making abilities and/ or may not have access to HIV protective-barrier devices. Further, infected people with few economic resources at their disposal usually are not organized or politically active.

Given these problems, the nurse assumes an active advocacy role. The nurse also has an important role to play in preventing the development of AIDS hysteria in the community. As both a professional and member of the community, the nurse can help others understand the facts about HIV/AIDS and alleviate their fears.

As an advocate for the person with HIV/AIDS, the nurse can facilitate access to a broad range of services needed by the person with HIV/AIDS and his or her family members, friends, and, if appropriate, school officials and work colleagues. These services include, but are not limited to, access to entitlement programs, home care, residential care, discharge planning, community referrals, and "buddy" programs (person-to-person assistance).

Where bureaucratic obstacles exist, the nurse as advocate provides assistance to facilitate the HIV-positive person's access to necessary resources. Advocating on behalf of persons with HIV/AIDS includes both assuring access to therapeutic regimens and supporting HIV-positive individuals who, having considered the options, decline to avail themselves of such therapies. The nurse also may assist those individuals who wish to integrate such therapies as acupuncture, meditation, and relaxation exercises into their health care regimen.

The nurse who works with persons with HIV/AIDS is in the best position to appreciate their needs and concerns. Using this knowledge base, the nurse takes action at the policy development level within the health care system and the community to assure that needed services are developed or shaped into an appropriate form. The nurse can facilitate activities so that collective grievances are addressed or resolved by judicial or legislative action, injurious practices are revised or discontinued, and the care system becomes responsive to those it was intended to serve.

The Cost of Care

A recent study of 10 American cities found that the estimated lifetime cost of medical care for a person with HIV infection is $119,000. The estimated cost of care from HIV infection until the development of AIDS is $50,000, and from AIDS until death is $69,000. One factor that has influenced the cost of care has been the length of hospitalization in acute-care facilities. The average length of acute-care hospitalization for an HIV-infected person with one of the opportunistic diseases of AIDS is 19 days per year, compared with 6.5 days per year for people with all other diseases (Hellinger 1993).

Many people with AIDS end up being hospitalized three or four times with exacerbations of the disease and development of multiple opportunistic infections (Jenna 1987; Sedaka 1986). These figures may change as more treatments and preventive strategies for complications are provided on an outpatient basis. However, costs increase as treatments improve and individuals live longer. Therefore, given improvements in the prognosis and treatment of HIV-infected people, it is difficult to predict the impact of these changes on the cost of care.

A significant factor influencing the cost of care is whether community-based subacute services and resources exist. In some areas, persons with HIV/AIDS have been forced to remain in acute-care facilities because of a lack of appropriate or adequate community-based support services, such as outpatient treatment centers, home health care, hospice care, skilled nursing care, residential placement, personal/attendant care, and practical support resources.

A recent study documented that persons with HIV/AIDS receiving a case-management model of care (such as the one funded by the CARE Act) had significantly lower hospital charges than persons with HIV/AIDS receiving traditional health care (Sowell et al. 1992).

Through the CARE Act, all states and territories and highly affected cities receive funds to provide services to persons with HIV infection. To provide the resources necessary for lowering the inpatient costs of care for persons with HIV/AIDS, increased funding for the CARE Act is being sought in 1994.

Financing Health Care

Health care reform, when implemented, may help resolve many of the problems persons with HIV infection experience in financing their health care. In the meantime, health care financing is a critical issue for a large percentage of those with HIV/AIDS, and one that nurses, as policy makers and advocates, must address in order to assist HIV-positive individuals in obtaining health care.

In this section, private insurance coverage as well as Medicaid and Medicare coverage are considered, problems that may be encountered in obtaining or maintaining medical coverage are examined, and mechanisms the nurse can utilize to assist the person with HIV/AIDS in resolving the problems are outlined. The problems of health care and personal care needs that are not financed by health insurance also are discussed.

A number of factors contribute to persons with HIV/AIDS having difficulty in obtaining financing for their health care. First, the primary source of health insurance in the United States is employers, causing problems when a person no longer can work. Second, a number of insurance loopholes have been used by private insurance companies to discriminate against persons with HIV/AIDS (Jackson 1992). Third, the alternative forms of health care coverage in this country—Medicaid and Medicare—have strict qualification criteria, which many of those with HIV/AIDS do not meet. For example, an adult must be disabled and indigent to qualify for Medicaid, or must be disabled for at least two years or over 65 years old to qualify for Medicare.

Persons with HIV/AIDS utilize a wide range of sources for health care coverage. In a 1992 national survey of persons with HIV/AIDS, nearly half the respondents were covered by private insurance, nearly 10 percent by Medicare, 17 percent by Medicaid, and the rest by a variety of sources, including free health care and paying all costs out-of-pocket.

Of those with private health insurance, over 10 percent paid for individual policies, nearly 20 percent had health insurance paid for by an employer, and another 20 percent either shared the cost of premiums with an employer or paid entirely for group insurance coverage themselves (National Association of People with AIDS 1992). Because responses were obtained through medical and community-based services, this survey probably under-represents disenfranchised persons with HIV/AIDS who have no health care coverage and, therefore, are not obtaining services at all.

The option of private insurance coverage for persons with HIV/AIDS appears to be decreasing. In a Philadelphia study of persons with HIV/AIDS, the percentage with private health care insurance decreased from 51.9 percent in 1988 to 28.6 percent in 1991. While some of this change reflects the growing incidence of AIDS among poor and underserved populations, adjusting for demographic and behavioral characteristics did not remove the statistically significant drop in private health care insurance (Fife and McAnaney 1993).

The amount of protection for persons with HIV/AIDS from insurance policy exclusion or from the loss or reduction of insurance coverage varies widely. Regulation of insurance companies differs according to the type of coverage and state regulations. Two kinds of health coverage are employment-based:

1. the traditional group health insurance plan, which is provided by a commercial health insurance company regulated by the state; and,
2. employer self-insurance, which is provided by the employer, with the pool of employees comprising the risk pool.

Commercial health insurance companies are regulated by the state, and some states have explicit protections for persons with HIV/AIDS. Even in such states, self-insured companies are exempt from state regulations (Jackson 1992).

There is a wide range of mechanisms that are used to avoid covering health care costs for persons with HIV/AIDS. Companies actually have been able to exclude HIV-related health care costs from their health plans, place caps on the total amount of coverage for HIV-related costs, and restrict coverage for all prescription drugs or uses of drugs that are not explicitly listed by the Federal Drug Administration (FDA). Companies also have refused to provide coverage to individuals or groups of people based on a perception that they might be at risk for HIV infection (Jackson 1992).

The HIV-infected individual may or may not have recourse against these types of exclusions according to his or her coverage and the specific state regulations. Nurses often can refer persons with HIV/AIDS to local AIDS service organizations, many of which have social or legal services departments that can assist an individual in determining whether he or she can contest an insurance company's actions. In addition, a book recently published by the American Civil Liberties Union (ACLU 1993) describes successful and unsuccessful litigation of specific cases, and outlines possible legal remedies, including federal statutes and regulations, for individuals experiencing this type of discrimination (Durham 1991; Jackson 1992).

The Americans with Disabilities Act of 1990 has increased federal protection against discrimination facing persons with HIV/AIDS (see Appendix F). Although the act is less than clear about whether insurance coverage is protected, it is still a landmark piece of legislation in protecting the HIV-infected person from employment discrimination.

If a person with HIV/AIDS does have private insurance, he or she can now maintain that coverage when no longer able to work. The Consolidated Omnibus Budget Reconciliation Act (COBRA) of 1985 requires most employers to provide departing employees with continuation of their health insurance policies, and requires insurance companies to offer conversion from group to individual coverage when the continuation period expires. If an individual resigns because of a disability, the continuation period is 29 months, which is long enough to satisfy the waiting period required for people with disabilities to qualify for Medicare. In many cases, the real problem is maintaining the insurance premiums. In such cases, some states provide funding to help maintain private insurance premiums through either the CARE Act or Medicaid.

It is virtually impossible for an already identified HIV-infected individual to obtain a private individual health insurance policy that covers HIV-related health care costs at a reasonable premium. The only way for an HIV-infected person to obtain private insurance is through a work-related group insurance plan. A disabled person with HIV disease who has lost private insurance coverage either must qualify for Medicaid or Medicare, obtain free health care at a public clinic, or pay out-of-pocket for all medical costs. In their case-management activities, therefore, it is critical for nurses to assist those persons with HIV/AIDS who are covered by private insurance to maintain their policies, utilizing COBRA regulations and whatever funding sources are available to pay the premiums.

Medicare is the federally funded health care plan for those who have paid a sufficient amount into Social Security during their working years, and who are over the age of 65 years or who have been disabled for at least two years. After receiving Social Security Disability Insurance for two years, a person automatically qualifies for Medicare. Unfortunately, most people with AIDS do not live long enough after becoming fully disabled to benefit from Medicare coverage. It has been estimated that Medicare pays only 2.5 percent of the national AIDS-related health care costs, compared with 26 percent covered by Medicaid (Shacknai 1992).

Medicaid is the federal health care plan for totally indigent people. Although the program implementation differs from state to state, the income limit for eligibility in 1990 was $386 per month, with additional assets of only $2,000 allowed, besides ownership of a car and the house the person lived in. For a person with no health care coverage and high costs that must be paid out-of-pocket, the process of becoming sufficiently indigent to qualify for Medicaid is inevitable. Because the processes documenting indigent status and disability for persons with HIV/AIDS are complicated and time-consuming, nurses may refer potential applicants to the hospital or home-care AIDS coordinator, or to a local AIDS service organization that provides assistance in qualifying for benefits.

In addition to documenting indigent status, a person with HIV infection must prove 100 percent disability according to Social Security Administration guidelines in order to qualify for Medicaid, unless he or she has a diagnosed case of AIDS, which confers automatic disability status. While the diagnosis of AIDS is fairly straightforward (see Appendix C), the documentation of disability for the person with HIV infection who does not have a diagnosis is much more complicated. The Social Security Administration guidelines for HIV-related disability claims were revised in June 1993 and are much improved, though still complex (Keller 1993).

None of the health care financing options discussed in this section provides coverage for all of the needs of a person with HIV/AIDS. Services such as home care, long-term care, hospice care, and the myriad of direct support services—such as transportation, child care, housing, home delivery of meals, and substance abuse treatment—that enable a disabled person to obtain health care or to function in the community often are not covered or are inadequately covered by private insurance, Medicare, and Medicaid.

Privately-funded AIDS service organizations emerged early in the pandemic to address many of these needs. Additionally, coordinated programs of service delivery were initiated in the mid-1980s through the funding of community demonstration projects in major cities by the federal government and the Robert Wood Johnson Foundation. The concept of case management for persons with HIV/AIDS emerged, with nurses playing a primary role. Finally, the CARE Act of 1990 has enabled coordinated service delivery systems to be funded in all 50 states and in cities with high numbers of AIDS cases.

Each city and state has different services available to augment the health care system for persons with HIV/AIDS, and the nurse can assist HIV-positive individuals to address the problems of health care financing by identifying the available resources. For some, referral to specific AIDS service agencies may be sufficient. For others, referral directly to the Social Security Administration or to the local Medicaid office may be necessary. If so, it is important to know the names of AIDS-knowledgeable workers in these agencies, and to refer persons with HIV/AIDS specifically to those workers.

In addition, the nurse can provide assistance to those who are attempting to apply for benefits by knowing how to facilitate completion of the required forms. Qualifying as disabled, for example, requires the completion of forms designating levels of ability. Health care providers unfamiliar with the terminology and concepts of these forms may be unable to provide adequate assistance to a person with HIV/AIDS.

Educating Persons with HIV/AIDS

Nurses have excelled at providing the information and support necessary to help persons with HIV/AIDS make the most appropriate decisions about their treatment. Even though there currently is no cure for HIV infection, drug and treatment protocols that often are effective in treating opportunistic disease, alleviating symptoms, and prolonging life are available.

It is the primary care provider's responsibility to provide information about treatment choices and experimental drug protocols. The nurse can augment decision making by providing information so that the person with HIV/AIDS is able to make informed choices about the direction and extent of treatment.

In addition, nontraditional therapies—such as visualization (mental imagery), relaxation exercises, and acupuncture—can be used as adjuncts to the more traditional therapies. Providing options to persons with HIV/AIDS facilitates their ability to live with symptomatic HIV disease. Knowledge about various therapies and referral resources enhances the nurse's ability to meet the needs of the person with HIV/AIDS.

Additionally, knowledge about durable power of attorney and the ability to discuss this option, including resuscitation code status, is essential for providing meaningful interventions for the person with HIV/AIDS. The nurse's commitment to the fundamental ethical principle of respect for the individual prepares the nurse to provide a supportive environment for the HIV-positive person's decision-making process, and to accept that person's right to self-determination.

The nurse's ethical responsibility is to educate and encourage the person with HIV/AIDS to share the diagnosis with his or her sexual or needle-sharing partners. The nurse can provide the skill-building techniques to empower him or her to do so, or can offer to assist in telling the partners. In addition, providing education that results in behavior changes to prevent further transmission of the HIV virus is a major responsibility of all health care workers.

Seropositive women should be informed and counseled regarding the potential for perinatal or other transmission (e.g., through breast milk) of the HIV virus, and should be provided with contraceptive information and contraception, if desired. Many seropositive women choose to become pregnant, and many women only discover that they are seropositive when they are offered HIV testing during prenatal care. The right of the seropositive woman to self-determination regarding whether to complete or terminate a pregnancy must be respected.

Educating the Family

Members of the family support system for the person with HIV/AIDS may have many fears and misconceptions about HIV transmission and the disease process, including fears of contagion through casual contact or through the provision of personal care. The nurse should address these fears through clear, straightforward teaching, and by acting as an appropriate role model.

Members of the family support system also may be unsure of how to relate to the HIV-positive person's diagnosis, debilitation, and potential death. This is an area in which ongoing teaching and counseling by the nurse can provide invaluable assistance to the family in coping with the crisis of this illness.

Family relationships will undergo strain, not only because of the life-threatening, chronic nature of the person's illness, but also because of the dramatic role changes that can occur as the person with HIV/AIDS becomes disabled. Financial strain also may add to family tension.

The person with HIV/AIDS is frequently reluctant to tell his or her family the diagnosis. The nurse may be able to provide support to the HIV-positive individual to enable him or her to tell the family, or can perhaps assist in telling them.

Partner Notification

The person who is HIV-infected should be encouraged to inform anyone he or she may have exposed to HIV, either through sexual contact or through sharing needles during drug use. If the person with HIV/AIDS has a spouse or steady sexual partner, informing the partner of his or her HIV status or AIDS diagnosis takes on an added dimension, particularly if the partner's HIV status is negative or unknown. The person with HIV/AIDS may fear the partner's anger, rejection, or even physical attack. The nurse can encourage and support the person with HIV/AIDS to tell his or her partner.

Partners should be made aware of the HIV status or AIDS diagnosis for several reasons. First, the partner is at risk and needs to be tested to determine whether he or she is also infected. (Condoms should be used if the couple subsequently chooses to engage in sexual contact.) Second, sharing this information with an intimate partner will ease the emotional burden associated with keeping the diagnosis a secret. Coping with the crisis together often can strengthen relationships.

Voluntary and confidential partner notification is currently available through all state and territorial health departments. The nurse can refer HIV-infected persons to this service for assistance in notifying their previous sexual or needle-sharing partners that they have been exposed to HIV. In some states, all persons with a positive HIV antibody test must be reported to the health department, and the partner notification program then contacts the individuals, usually after obtaining permission from the infected person's treatment provider.

Trained health department personnel can assist HIV-positive persons in notifying their sexual or drug-using partners themselves (*patient referral model*), or the HIV-positive person can give the names of his or her partners to the health department official (*provider referral model*). The official then contacts all of the partners, saying that an HIV-infected individual (whose name is never divulged) has identified them as a sexual or needle-sharing contact. Confidential HIV counseling and testing will then be offered by the health department to the contacted partners.

ANA supports the availability of voluntary and confidential partner notification services for HIV-positive individuals (see Appendix A). ANA also endorses the concept of an ethical responsibility to disclose otherwise confidential information about probable HIV exposure when the person with HIV/AIDS fails to uphold his or her duty to protect others by preventing transmission of the infecting agent, but only when specific criteria have been met and documented (see Appendix A). Beyond this, nurses should be aware of local or state laws before taking it upon themselves to inform partners.

Under the following circumstances, it is the nurse's ethical responsibility to disclose otherwise confidential information to a known third party (usually the steady sexual partner of an HIV-infected person):

- the nurse is the primary provider of health care and knows of an identifiable third party at risk;
- the nurse believes that there is a significant risk of harm (through sexual or blood-to-blood contact) to the third party;
- the identified person with HIV/AIDS has been urged to notify the at-risk partner and has refused to, or is considered to be unreliable in his or her ability to notify the partner; or,
- the infected person has been counseled regarding the provider's intent to notify (see Appendix A).

Partner notification should be undertaken only by a nurse or health care worker who is skilled in the biological and psychosocial aspects of HIV infection. Providers need to be well prepared in counseling specific to HIV infection and according to appropriate community standards in order to inform unsuspecting partners of probable HIV exposure. Informing unsuspecting partners or contacts may create disturbing situations requiring the availability of a wide range of psychological, legal, social, family, and emergency services. Providers must be aware of the applicable laws regarding the notification of public health officials and contact or partner notification requirements in their jurisdiction. Liability issues related to notification and counseling require constant monitoring.

6

Work Force Issues

Basic Nursing Education

In the academic setting, nurse educators must address the multitude of issues related to HIV infection to prepare students to deal effectively with the needs of their patients in the practice setting. Appropriate HIV-related content and competencies should be incorporated at all levels, from basic to graduate education.

Some of the areas of curriculum development that may require strengthening include:

- physiology of the immune system
- virology (especially concerning retroviruses)
- mechanisms of disease transmission
- student values clarification
- diversity of ethnicities and life styles among people with HIV/AIDS (including sexual orientation and substance use)
- psychosocial issues such as death and dying
- ethical and legal issues
- occupational safety issues
- the use of nontraditional therapies by people with HIV/AIDS, and
- the role of the nurse in primary health care and case management.

Because of the importance of the multidisciplinary team approach in providing services to persons with HIV/AIDS, the roles of the other members of the caregiving team, the family, and the physician—from inpatient to community-based settings—must be emphasized to students.

Nursing education also should include the development of skills in the following areas:
- initiating assessment procedures
- obtaining the sexual and intravenous drug-use history of the person with HIV/AIDS
- discussing the intimate aspects of the HIV-positive person's sexual behaviors
- working with the dual diagnosis of chemical dependency and HIV/AIDS
- advocating for the person with HIV/AIDS
- facilitating services
- understanding entitlements and health care financing, and
- counseling the newly diagnosed HIV-positive person, as well as the dying person with HIV/AIDS.

Academic programs must specifically address the diverse psychological and psychosocial needs of persons with HIV/AIDS. The nurse caring for HIV-positive individuals must be knowledgeable about the effects of the illness on the person's central nervous system and about the potentially impaired thinking and decision making that can subsequently affect behavior. Since dementia increasingly affects persons with AIDS, it is important for the nurse to be familiar with neuropsychiatric manifestations such as apathy, depression, memory loss, and motor deficits (Flaskerud 1987; McArthur and McArthur 1986).

The nurse must be prepared to assess the mental status of the person with HIV/AIDS for any significant changes in thought processes, affect, or behavior that might indicate functional psychological problems—often induced by the devastating levels of stress, change, and loss experienced by the person with HIV/AIDS. Skills in early recognition and timely referral for appropriate psychotherapeutic intervention are especially important in relation to common problematic socio-emotional responses such as guilt, shame, anxiety, fear, anger, denial, grief, and suicidal ideation.

Knowledge of the HIV-infected person's family and social system is essential and can enable the nurse to provide needed care to the person dealing with the almost inevitable disruption of significant social relationships and support systems, including the need to cope with social isolation, rejection, and/or prejudice.

Continuing Nursing Education

Because of the rapidly growing body of research and information related to HIV, continuing education is vital for the nurse practicing in administrative, policy, or clinical settings. Nursing management must facilitate ongoing HIV/AIDS education for all nurses, as well as support for those nurses caring for HIV-infected individuals.

Continuing education must address a variety of subjects, but four areas that require regular updating are:

1. epidemiology
2. HIV treatment research
3. HIV prevention research, and
4. prevention of HIV transmission in the health care setting.

Epidemiology updates are important for keeping nurses informed about the demographic characteristics of newly affected populations of people and the clinical course of the HIV disease in various populations. Nurses require this information for the assessment of all persons with HIV/AIDS, for HIV prevention education, for recognition of early manifestations of the HIV disease process, and for early intervention in prophylaxis and treatment of opportunistic diseases.

Updates on treatment research are critical because new drugs, including antivirals, are constantly being developed and approved. Nurses need to be able to administer and monitor newly approved treatments properly, and to enable persons with HIV/AIDS to access clinical trials.

Updates on prevention research are pivotal in stemming the increasing tide of HIV-infected people. Nurses are on the front line of health care provision and must be adept at risk assessment, counseling, and intervention.

Updates on the prevention of HIV transmission in the health care setting are vital for nurses to practice effectively and safely. They need to be kept informed about epidemiological research on the risks of occupational exposure, as well as about research and the development of equipment that minimizes occupational exposure. In addition, nurses need to understand the OSHA regulations regarding prevention of the transmission of bloodborne pathogens (see Appendix E). Nurses require updates on such information as changes in the surveillance definition of AIDS, additional legal protections for persons with HIV/AIDS, and new community resources (see Appendix B).

Nurses who are actively caring for persons with HIV/AIDS need more than information—they need support. The care of persons with HIV infection and their families is an intense and difficult challenge. Nurses address the health, psychosocial, educational, and resource needs of the person with HIV/AIDS and his or her family. If the HIV-positive person has problems such as substance abuse, homelessness, or lack of a means of support, case management may require a great deal of counseling, as well as interaction with other agencies.

The chronicity and terminal nature of HIV disease results in repeated and extensive hospitalizations, ongoing home care, and long-term or hospice care. Over this period of time, staff often become emotionally involved with the HIV-positive patients for whom they care. The development and implementation of programs that support and address the needs of caregivers are vital for the continuing delivery of quality care. Programs such as ongoing education, staff support groups, and regular time off can assist in alleviating the fears of nurses and preventing burnout (Bennett 1987; Brown and Brown 1988; Jenna 1987).

Risk Reduction

For nurses, the greatest risk of exposure to HIV involves injury during the handling of sharps. The current known risk for becoming occupationally infected with HIV after a percutaneous exposure to blood containing HIV is approximately 0.3 percent. Other risks involve direct contact through open cuts, and splashing eyes, nose, or mouth with blood during care of and procedures with HIV-infected patients.

ANA supports the consistent and strict use of universal precautions by the health care provider (see Appendix D), and also supports other risk-reduction strategies that require administrative or institutional implementation, such as the availability of proven safety measures, the standardization of methods to ensure equipment is safe, and the continued evaluation and modification of work practices to assure optimum safety in the workplace (see Appendix A).

Strategies for reducing the risk of exposure to bloodborne pathogens, including HIV can be classified into three categories:
1. engineering controls
2. work practices, and
3. the use of personal protective equipment.

These categories define a hierarchy of strategies. Engineering controls are the best line of defense for protection of the nurse, and work practices are the second best line of defense. Personal protective equipment, the third best line of defense, only protects against the kinds of exposures that are least likely to result in transmission of infectious agents. It must be understood that the efficacy of engineering controls and safe work practices is dependent on their consistent use and application in the work setting by nurses.

With engineering controls being the first line of defense against occupational exposure to bloodborne pathogens, the workplace will continue to become more technologically advanced. Many nurses intuitively resist barriers between the care provider and the patient, as documented by studies of nurses (Gerberding 1992) failing to observe simple barrier precautions (the use of personal protective equipment) such as gloves when drawing blood. Engineering controls hold out the promise of removing the need for barriers by eliminating potential hazards in the first place.

Work practice controls reduce the likelihood of exposure by altering the way a task is performed (e.g., using a one-handed scoop technique when it is essential to recap a used needle). Work practice controls can address many situational issues related to the time certain risky tasks are performed. For example, data from the occupational health literature suggest that individuals may be most injury-prone at the end of a shift, when working either a double-shift or overtime, or after transfer to an unfamiliar area, especially if orientation is lacking.

Personal protective equipment includes gloves, gowns, eye protection, masks or face shields, and other garments intended to reduce the likelihood of blood or body fluids contaminating the skin, clothing, eyes, or mucous membranes. Protective equipment has received a great deal of attention, even though it only addresses the types of exposure risks that are far less likely to result in the transmission of infectious agents than are puncture or sharps injuries, which are better prevented through engineering and work practice controls.

While the nurse has a moral responsibility in most instances to provide care to all persons with HIV/AIDS, regardless of diagnosis, he or she also has the right to a safe work environment with reasonable and adequate protection from occupational exposure to HIV and other bloodborne pathogens. In 1992, the OSHA Standard on Occupational Exposure to Bloodborne Pathogens went into effect (see Appendix E). Under the standard, hospitals and other health care employers are required to develop and implement plans to protect employees from exposure to bloodborne pathogens, including HIV.

In addition to supporting the OSHA standard, there is a critical need for 1) aggressive development of new protective devices, 2) research on the effectiveness of these devices in protecting health care workers from injury and exposure to blood, and 3) dissemination of information on effective devices so they can be implemented in the workplace.

ANA supports immediate systematic research and evaluation studies of devices and equipment intended to reduce the risk of injury from sharps, and of personal protective equipment designed to reduce exposure risk. In addition, as soon as safety devices are proven effective, they must be available in all appropriate settings, and proper training concerning their use must be provided. Necessary protective equipment and supplies—such as gloves, goggles, masks, gowns, Ambu bags, and mouthpieces—must be readily available and accessible to all staff members.

Written protocols that specify appropriate infection control measures must be developed and implemented in all health care settings. All staff must receive regular training in universal infection precautions, prevention of the transmission of bloodborne pathogens, the use of protective equipment, and the documentation of accidents involving exposure to blood.

Occupational Exposure to HIV

The Centers for Disease Control and Prevention are conducting national surveillance of occupational exposure to HIV in an effort to define more precisely the level of risk of HIV infection in the health care setting. In a recent report regarding this study, the seroconversion rates following occupational exposure to HIV were reported for occupationally exposed health care workers. Four of the 1,103 workers who experienced percutaneous exposure seroconverted, resulting in an HIV seroconversion rate of 0.35 percent. None of the 75 workers enrolled in the study—who experienced mucous membrane exposure—seroconverted (Tokars et al. 1993).

As of June 1993, the CDC had received reports of 37 documented cases of HIV infection acquired through occupational transmission among health care workers. Of these, 13 are nurses. In addition, there are 78 reports of *possible* occupational transmission, of which 15 involve nurses. Possible transmission is distinguished from documented transmission by the fact that in the latter, HIV seronegativity was demonstrated immediately after the occupational exposure, followed by HIV seroconversion (Centers for Disease Control 1993a).

The surveillance of occupational HIV exposure cannot be regarded as complete for a number of reasons, ranging from lack of awareness of the need to report to fear of reporting exposure. However, good evidence from the AIDS surveillance demonstrates that most HIV infections, and therefore AIDS, are not a result of occupational exposure. As of September 1988, a total of 61,929 adults with AIDS on whom occupational information was available had been reported to the CDC. Of these, 3,182 (5.1 percent) reported being employed in a health care setting. Of these health care workers with AIDS, 95 percent reported a high-risk behavior, while the means of HIV transmission to the other 5 percent was undetermined at that time (Centers for Disease Control 1989).

While we have no further information on the 5 percent of health care workers whose means of HIV infection was undetermined, most investigations of individuals with no identified risk result in their being classified into an existing risk category. As of June 1993, of the 10,718 reported AIDS cases, with no risk identified, that were investigated, 94 percent were reclassified into reportable risk categories, while .07 percent ($n = 8$) were identified as health care workers who developed AIDS after a documented occupational exposure to HIV-infected blood (Centers for Disease Control 1993a).

The CDC has developed guidelines for the management of health care workers following occupational exposure to HIV (see Appendix G). A comprehensive post-exposure program should be in place in all health care settings to ensure that employees who are possibly exposed to bloodborne pathogens receive accurate information, immediate evaluation, and prophylactic interventions, counseling, and supportive care. These procedures should be considered the standard of care by any health care agency. ANA encourages prompt access to confidential post-exposure evaluations, counseling, and follow-up by knowledgeable clinicians (see Appendix A).

The nurse who experiences an occupational exposure to blood during the course of work requires post-exposure services (counseling, testing, education, treatment, and prophylaxis). Support services may be necessary for both nurse and family members throughout the 6- to 12-month post-exposure monitoring period. The nurse who seroconverts requires ongoing medical care, and should be guaranteed workers' compensation benefits and continued health insurance coverage (see Appendix A).

HIV-Positive Health Care Providers

In a 1989 study to identify what percentage of persons with AIDS were health care workers, 5.1 percent reported being employed in health care settings. An equal number of persons with HIV infection are likely to work in health care settings, meaning that there undoubtedly are many health care workers who are HIV-infected (Centers for Disease Control 1989).

A great deal of controversy surrounds the issue of HIV-infected health care providers, particularly since the case of the woman who acquired AIDS following treatment by an HIV-infected dentist (Centers for Disease Control 1991d). The only risk of HIV transmission from nurse to patients would involve a nurse's blood entering a patient's body if the nurse was injured during an exposure-prone invasive procedure, such as abdominal surgery.

Nurses who know they have a transmissible bloodborne infection should voluntarily avoid exposure-prone invasive procedures that have been epidemiologically linked to HIV or other bloodborne infection transmission. In addition, the nurse has a duty to report the exposure of a patient to bloodborne infection (see Appendix A).

Public fear has resulted in ongoing requests that all health care workers be tested for HIV infection, and that those found to be HIV-positive be removed from the health care setting, or that at least their patients be informed of their HIV status. As early as 1988, ANA opposed the routine testing of health care workers and supported the HIV-infected nurse's right to confidentiality and protection from workplace discrimination (see Appendix A).

The removal of HIV-positive nurses from *routine practice* would be a profound loss of human resources from the profession, and is epidemiologically unnecessary. To require HIV-infected health care workers to disclose their HIV status to patients as a condition of practice would be an unnecessary and harmful breach of individual privacy, and would provide no protection to the patient.

The use of universal precautions and strict infection control procedures are the means by which nurse-to-patient as well as patient-to-nurse transmission of HIV infection can be eliminated. Therefore, the presence of HIV infection alone does not constitute a basis for nurses to withdraw from their practices. The circumstances of each HIV-infected nurse should be evaluated on a case-by-case basis relative to the extent to which procedures need to be limited.

Adherence to universal precautions and strict infection control procedures would eliminate all but the rarest cases of transmission. Furthermore, it must be emphasized that the most likely transmission route of bloodborne infection is from patient to nurse, *not* from nurse to patient.

HIV-infected nurses currently in the work force are an important and valuable resource to society, and should be supported in continuing to work as long as possible. In accordance with the Americans with Disabilities Act, working conditions should accommodate such nurses who choose to continue working—by implementing variable working hours, for instance, or a less physically strenuous position within the institution, to compensate for fatigue or decreased mobility.

HIV-infected nurses also benefit from support groups including other HIV-infected nurses. AIDS service organizations in large cities may offer this sort of service. State nurses associations are establishing support systems for members who are HIV-positive and confronting personal and professional challenges and tragedies. In addition, nursing continues to investigate workers' compensation provisions and to improve such benefits through legislative action.

Economic Issues

Discussions of the AIDS pandemic inevitably turn to economic issues. The loss of increasing numbers of young people from the work force in the midst of their most productive years is a heavy economic and human resource loss. The large number of disabled, acutely and chronically ill, and terminally ill persons with HIV/AIDS disease places a growing burden on health and social systems.

Inevitably, the intense psychosocial and physical needs of persons with HIV/AIDS, the needs of health care providers who must be trained to address these issues appropriately, and the need for implementation of universal precautions and engineering controls against bloodborne disease in the health care setting all have a significant economic impact on health care institutions.

The issue of worker protection also introduces considerations of economic concern. The training of staff in universal precautions requires resources. The use of engineering controls to protect health workers can be expected to require expenditures of funds, and ANA urges that financing mechanisms be explored to assure that cost does not limit the availability of proven safety devices (see Appendix A). The development of services to manage potential occupational exposure to HIV requires staff training and management time to develop protocols, and the provision of the necessary counseling and support services, if needed, is an additional expense.

The risk of occupational exposure to bloodborne pathogens, although very small, may be a factor in insurance carriers covering health care workers and raising their rates. Monitoring the costs of health coverage for health care workers will continue to be important.

Attempts have been made to address the economic impact of the pandemic on the health care system. The CARE Act is an effort on the part of the federal government to decrease the economic impact of HIV/AIDS on state and local health care systems. In addition to establishing measures such as the financing of direct services and ongoing insurance coverage for persons with HIV infection, the CARE Act establishes mechanisms for comprehensive and coordinated services to be provided to HIV-infected individuals, with the goal of decreasing the need for long and expensive hospital stays.

Nurses have assumed an increasingly important role in the provision of services to persons with HIV/AIDS. Nursing supports this expanded role for the nurse as the central, coordinating figure in the provision of primary health care. Health care reform with access to primary health care will help reduce the economic impact of the pandemic on the health care system through the cost-effective utilization of nurses and nursing services to provide quality care to those with HIV/AIDS and their families.

7

Research

The Nursing Research Agenda

Nursing research provides the scientific foundation for interventions that are effective in enhancing the health and well-being of all members of our society. Recognizing the significant contributions that nursing research can provide to the growing body of knowledge about HIV infection and related issues, the National Institute for Nursing Research (NINR) at the National Institutes of Health (NIH) convened the Conference on Nursing Research Priorities in 1988. The process of developing NINR research priorities represents the input of nurse scientists throughout the United States.

Each of these priorities was implemented through intensive review of the state-of-the-science by a multidisciplinary priority expert panel, through specific recommendations by the panel for the most essential research to be funded by NINR, and through an announcement in the NIH *Guide for Grants and Contracts* of NINR's specific interest, resulting in applications to be funded in the announced area of interest.

One of the seven nursing research priorities identified at the conference was "HIV Infection: Prevention and Care." At a second conference in November 1992, HIV-related research was again selected as one of the five research priorities for NINR during the next five years. In 1996, the priority will be "Effectiveness of Nursing Interventions in HIV/AIDS," which will:

Assess the effectiveness of biobehavioral nursing interventions to foster health-promoting behaviors of individuals at risk for

HIV/AIDS, and of biobehavioral interventions to ameliorate the effects of illness in individuals who are already infected. The focus is on individuals of different cultural backgrounds—especially women. The need to incorporate biobehavioral markers is noted (National Institute for Nursing Research 1993).

The need for HIV-related nursing research has been considered in a number of areas for nurses in practice. Some examples are found in Table 1.

Nursing research focusing on the prevention of viral transmission needs to address the question of how to motivate individuals to change health-threatening behaviors. Are certain types of behaviors associated with a reduction in immune competence and the onset

TABLE 1

Examples of Nursing Practice Research Needed

CARE PROVIDERS	NURSING RESEARCH FOCUS
Hospital Nurse	The prevention of viral transmission.
Outpatient Clinic Nurse	The teaching of patients with cognitive deficits and outcomes of psychosocial interventions.
School Nurse	Educational interventions that are effective in changing behaviors.
College Health Nurse	Motivation for changing health-threatening behaviors.
Occupational Health Nurse	Preventive education with regard to HIV/AIDS.
Community Health Nurse	The role of the family in supporting the HIV-infected family member.
Public Health Nurse	The integration of patients in community settings.
Home Health Nurse	Clients who receive case-management services and those who do not.
Hospice Nurse	The effects of self-determination and death on family survivors.
All Nurses	Attitudes, fears, and the affect on prevention activities and care delivery.

of symptoms? Are certain behaviors associated with an enhancement of immune competence?

Questions relating to the psychosocial support and teaching of HIV-infected individuals with cognitive deficits need to be addressed. Which strategies are most helpful at different levels of functioning? What is true "informed" consent? What is the difference in an HIV-infected person's knowledge levels and understanding of the disease process, treatment protocols, and research protocols when education is provided by nurses as compared with other health care providers?

There is a need to examine which educational interventions are most effective in changing behaviors and which interventions are appropriate for different health care settings. Demonstration programs are needed in various settings, such as the inner city; schools; prisons; industrial, commercial, and educational work sites; churches, synagogues, mosques, and other places of worship; and clinics and community health centers. These programs should target such population groups as minorities, the homeless, children, teens, pregnant women, homosexual men, heterosexual men and women, and injection drug users.

Research also is needed as to what attitudes among nurses create obstacles to the effective implementation of educational strategies, and what barriers to prevention education exist in health care settings. Research is needed on the HIV-related attitudes and fears of nurses and other health care workers. How prevalent are homophobic and other prejudicial attitudes? What effect do these attitudes have on prevention activities and the care of persons with HIV infection?

Another area for research is the effectiveness of the health care industry in implementing universal infection-control precautions for handling blood and body fluids. Are health care workers effectively educated on practicing in accordance with infection control precautions? Are the materials to implement universal blood and body fluid precautions readily available? Which disinfecting solutions are effective in the prevention of HIV transmission? Are nurses providing humane care to individuals with HIV infection without endangering their own health? What impact is AIDS having on recruitment into the nursing profession, particularly by health care institutions in specific geographic areas?

Areas for scientific inquiry into treatment are varied. There is a serious need for research with injection drug users. The problems associated with HIV should serve as a catalyst for additional research into investigating new approaches to the problem of addiction. Questions surrounding the efficacy of HIV transmission prevention measures, such as needle exchange programs, need to be addressed.

Nurses in direct HIV/AIDS care can contribute significantly to nursing research and the improvement of care to HIV-infected and potentially infected persons by collaborating with their nursing research colleagues. In their daily work, nurses make observations and use a repertoire of modalities with an impact on AIDS care that could generate important research questions. Recording observations for further discussion with colleagues can lead to the fruitful examination of important questions.

The researcher is interested in determining the relative value of different interventions in order to enhance nursing practice. Questions as to which nursing interventions facilitate response to therapy, and whether they are the treatment of opportunistic infections or of progressive neurological deterioration, are basic to the scientific development of nursing modalities. Using qualitative research methodologies, descriptive studies of less-understood phenomena—such as hope—are essential and should be encouraged.

The need for nursing research is obvious. The need for the funding of research by nurses is equally clear. Current federal legislation gives limited support to research on nursing interventions, nursing demonstration programs, and the organization of care for persons with HIV infection. Until this is changed, nursing's potential to effect solutions for problems related to AIDS will not be realized.

The Research Impact of Persons with HIV/AIDS

Persons with HIV/AIDS have caused significant changes in how research is conducted in the United States. Advocacy groups have stimulated changes in research procedures, making potentially effective drugs available much more quickly.

Pressure from women's advocacy groups has caused significant improvement in the availability of clinical trials to women of child-bearing age, a group that traditionally has been excluded because of the potential to affect pregnancy and possibly endanger the fetus. Women's groups also have pressured the government to investigate the gynecological effects of HIV disease and the gynecological effects of treatments. These areas were not well investigated during the first 10 years of the pandemic.

Persons with HIV/AIDS as Participants in Research

Persons with HIV infection and populations heavily affected by HIV infection have eagerly been subjects of HIV-related research, ranging from biomedical to behavioral. Because so many HIV-infected people participate in research, the nurse has a responsibility to understand the ethical guidelines and standards for clinical and behavioral research.

While it is important to ensure that persons with HIV/AIDS have reasonable access to participation in research, it is even more important to ensure that their rights are respected while they are participating. Individuals with HIV/AIDS are vulnerable and easily subject to coercion. All research participants must receive adequate information, give informed consent, have their confidentiality maintained, and understand that they can withdraw from the research at any time. In addition, nurses must be attuned to signs and symptoms of the patient's condition that may be related to the research, and must be able to explain these to the HIV-infected individual so that he or she can choose to continue or stop participating.

Nurses' Participation in Clinical/ Investigative Drug Trials

NIH is conducting national multicenter HIV/AIDS clinical and investigative drug trials. Nurses are playing key roles in the development, management, and implementation of these studies. There are opportunities for the nurse to develop and use research skills while participating in protocol development, proposal writing, study design, subject recruitment, randomization and treatment, data collection and analysis, and the summary and presentation of study results. During these processes, it is critical for the nurse to maintain the role of advocate, always acting in an informed manner for the interests of each individual person with HIV/AIDS, while still maintaining the integrity of the study.

Nurses' participation in and contributions to clinical studies should be acknowledged when study results are published and disseminated. Individual nurses who play key roles should insist that their names be included as appropriate. Nurses should be ever alert for opportunities to pursue answers to nursing questions as they work in collaboration with other members of the research team.

8

Nurses in the HIV/AIDS Political Process

Since the beginning of the HIV/AIDS pandemic, nurses have played significant roles in the political processes related to HIV/AIDS on federal, state, and local levels. The AIDS pandemic is a volatile issue with social, ethical, legal, economic, and health care ramifications. There have been fiery debates within governments (both legislative and executive branches) and health care institutions as legislation and policies are crafted and recrafted to address AIDS-related issues.

Nursing has contributed a valuable perspective to these debates and has helped to shape effective policies related to the care of persons with HIV/AIDS and the prevention of HIV infection. In addition to clinical expertise, nurses have a broad understanding of the needs of the whole person in society, and are thus able to contribute a well-balanced perspective to the development of public and health policy related to HIV/AIDS.

On the federal level, ANA has worked with other professional health associations, with health care and other coalitions, and with federal health agencies to protect the rights of persons with HIV infection, to advocate strong and effective prevention activities for continuing HIV/AIDS public and provider education, and to advocate for resources for care as well as research. For example, ANA supported both the Americans with Disabilities Act and the CARE Act.

On the state level, state nurses associations have participated in the development of legislation to protect persons with HIV/AIDS from discrimination, and have pressed for resources to develop pro grams for HIV prevention and care. They have opposed legislation that would infringe on the rights of nurses and persons with HIV infection, or that would be counterproductive to effective HIV education.

On the local level, nurses have participated in city-wide task forces and advisory groups, and have played key roles in the development of legislation, health department policy, and community-based plans for HIV education and care of HIV-infected persons. Nurses have played a primary role in the development of effective workplace policies to educate nurses about and protect them from exposure to HIV.

9

Challenges beyond the Year 2000

As we approach the year 2000, the number of persons with HIV/AIDS continues to increase, the impact of the pandemic on the health care system broadens, and the challenge to nursing becomes greater. The pandemic will demand an increasing amount of our nation's social and health resources in the coming decades.

As a profession, nursing will need to continue recruiting and preparing capable practitioners to ensure the ongoing provision of a competent, caring work force. The role of nursing in addressing the impact of the pandemic will continue to be significant, with nurses applying new technologies to HIV/AIDS care. With improvements in engineering controls, the risk of occupational exposure to bloodborne pathogens should decrease. Nurses will continue to meet broad needs for community and individual education, psychosocial support, coordination of care/case management, and treatment in a variety of institutional and community settings.

The challenge for prevention also will be significant. As new generations become sexually active, there will be an ongoing need to empower individuals to protect themselves from infection. This is particularly significant in light of increases in sexually transmitted diseases and drug use.

Today's society has a short-term attention span for "current issues." Interest in HIV/AIDS is already waning, as new social issues compete for our attention and our nation's limited resources. Creative approaches involving targeted messages will be needed to reach those who practice risky behaviors. Also, nurses will need to refine educational information to include more specific culturally-, behaviorally-, and sexually-oriented language, so that the people who need to be reached will respond to and understand the message. Medically technical information will need to be converted to street language if it is going to provide a clear message to diverse communities.

Nurses have firsthand experience with the stark, cold reality of HIV/AIDS disease on a daily basis. They must deal with the key, preexisting, deeply imbedded societal issues of inequity and discrimination. Nurses have strength, give hope, and listen and touch while providing nursing care. They will continue to be the force for change for prevention initiatives, quality care delivery, culturally sensitive perspectives, safer work environments, significant research, and strong advocacy for persons with HIV/AIDS.

ANA's Decade of HIV/AIDS Policies and Position Statements

A

The American Nurses Association (ANA) has been actively involved in the HIV/AIDS epidemic for over a decade, and continues to provide a leadership role for nursing and other health care professionals dealing with this major health problem. Throughout the course of the illness in the individual with HIV infection, nurses play a critical role in the creation and maintenance of support services for the client. Often young and facing death, individuals with HIV/AIDS come to the health care system with extraordinary physical, psychological, socioeconomic, and spiritual needs.

Because of nursing's focus on comprehensive care, the nursing profession, perhaps more than any other discipline, has been challenged to meet these needs. Nurses are in a unique position to provide leadership as a result of understanding the humanistic mandate to make health care accessible to all members of society, and are sensitive to the ethical dimensions of the nurse's role in the delivery of care, particularly in times of life-threatening, widespread illness. Unique to the profession of nursing is the ability to combine the latest scientific findings with the need for appropriate care and compassion for the client, in order to formulate policies ensuring the commitment of all in society to an ethos of mutual caring. As nurses, we can do no less.

The full text of the following position statements is available in the American Nurses Association's *Compendium of HIV/AIDS Position Statements, Policies, and Documents* (ANA 1993).

Care for At-Risk Populations, Independent of HIV/AIDS Status

Social Responsibility for Health Care Services to At-Risk Populations, 1982

The contents of this policy have been incorporated into subsequent policies and position statements.

Health Care for a Population at Risk, 1984 (updated 1985)

This position statement was incorporated into the 1991 position statements.

Regarding Risk vs. Responsibility in Providing Nursing Care, 1986

These concepts have been incorporated into many subsequent documents, and the intent is included in the 1991 position statements.

HIV Disease and Correctional Inmates, 1992

Federal, state, local, and juvenile correctional facilities house significant numbers of individuals who are at risk for HIV disease. Voluntary testing, strict application of universal precautions and CDC guidelines, education/counseling services, availability of protective devices, and confidentiality are important issues for nurses working in these settings. (Approved, September 1992.)

HIV Disease and Women, 1992

Heterosexual transmission of HIV/AIDS is increasingly being identified as the primary mode of transmission, and significant numbers of women now have the disease. Scientific knowledge of care that is culturally sensitive and relevant to the needs of women needs to be developed. (Approved, September 1992).

AIDS/HIV Disease in Socio-Culturally Diverse Populations, 1993

ANA supports the provision of skilled, knowledgeable, and compassionate nursing care that respects the client's conscience and integrity, cultural values, beliefs, relationships, and the right to make choices. Comprehensive educational programs that are culturally sensitive must be targeted to diverse population groups to assure that the HIV/AIDS pandemic is stopped in all communities. Continued political action and advocacy also is needed to ensure quality health for all. (Approved, April 1993).

HIV *Exposure from Rape/Sexual Assault*, 1993

Rape/sexual assault is a violent crime that affects adults (both women and men) and children. A person who survives rape/sexual assault is placed at risk for both psychological and physical trauma. Nurses believe that access to survivor-focused services, which include appropriate HIV testing and prophylactic treatment, should be available in health care settings. (Approved, April 1993.)

Needle Exchange and HIV, 1993

An increasing number of HIV/AIDS cases are related to injection drug use. Nurses support the availability of needle exchange programs that include adherence to public health and infection control guidelines, access to referral for treatment and rehabilitation services, and education about the transmission of HIV disease. (Approved, April 1993.)

Tuberculosis and HIV, 1993

Resurgence of tuberculosis (TB) and the identification of multidrug-resistant strains of tuberculosis (MDR-TB) have created a major U.S. health threat to all people, including those who are immuno-suppressed. Nurses believe that access is needed to essential TB testing, treatment, education, counseling, and follow-up services for the public and health care providers. (Approved, April 1993.)

The Public

Acquired Immune Deficiency Syndrome (AIDS), 1987

This policy, which appears in an informational report to the 1987 House of Delegates, has been incorporated into the 1991 position statements.

Access to Psychological and Psychosocial Nursing Care for AIDS Clients, 1988

The content of this policy has been incorporated into the 1991 position statements.

Education and Barrier Use for Sexually Transmitted Diseases (STDs) and HIV Infection, 1991

Nurses believe sexually transmitted diseases are a major health problem in the United States. ANA supports condom advertising in the mass media as a means of controlling and preventing the spread of sexually transmitted diseases. Further, ANA continues to work with the U.S. Public Health Service and other groups to educate the public on preventive measures. (Approved, September 1991.)

HIV Infection and U.S. Teenagers, 1991

The incidence of HIV infection among U.S. teenagers is increasing, and is clearly associated with increasing sexual activity among young men and women. Nurses believe that increased education about the risks of HIV infection, basic sex information (including the option of abstinence), and the essential features of safer sex practices should be a priority within school curricula targeting young people, and within community health nursing practice. Prevention strategies should include education about the risks of HIV infection and drug use, advertising and distribution of condoms to minors, and greater access by teenagers and college-age students to preventive health care services by qualified providers. (Approved, December 1991.)

Travel Restrictions for Persons with HIV/AIDS, 1991

ANA opposes the U.S. State Department policy that imposes travel restrictions on visitors with HIV/AIDS. ANA believes this policy is discriminatory and infringes upon the rights and dignity of individuals with HIV/AIDS. Further, ANA supports the enactment of federal legislation to revoke the current travel restrictions. (Approved, September 1991.)

AIDS *and the* Workplace

Recommendations for Preventing Transmission of HIV Infections in the Workplace, 1988

The content of this policy has been updated and incorporated into the 1991 "Position Statement on Personnel Policies and HIV in the Workplace."

AIDS *and the* Impact on Workplace Policies, 1987

The content of this policy has been updated and incorporated into the 1991 "Position Statement on Personnel Policies and HIV in the Workplace."

AIDS *and the* Continuing Impact on Workplace Policies, 1988

The content of this policy has been updated and incorporated into the 1991 "Position Statement on Personnel Policies and HIV in the Workplace."

Availability of Equipment and Safety Procedures to Prevent Transmission of Bloodborne Diseases, 1991

ANA urges immediate and ongoing research and evaluation of devices and equipment intended to reduce the risks of injury from sharps, and of personal protective equipment designed to reduce exposure. In order to reduce the risk of exposure to bloodborne pathogens, ANA supports the consistent and strict use of universal precautions, the availability of proven safety measures, the standardization of methods to assure that equipment is safe, and the continued evaluation and motivation of work practices to ensure optimum safety in the workplace. (Approved, September 1991.)

Post-Exposure Programs in the Event of Occupational Exposure to HIV/HBV, 1991

ANA encourages prompt access to confidential post-exposure evaluation, counseling, and follow-up by knowledgeable clinicians. These procedures should be considered the standard of care by any health care agency. A comprehensive post-exposure program should be in place to assure that employees receive accurate information, guidance, reassurance, and supportive care. (Approved, September 1991.)

Personnel Policies and HIV in the Workplace, 1991

ANA has a long-standing position of advocating for the rights of nurses in the workplace. The association supports the development of personnel policies that create a maximally safe and healthful environment for all workers, patients/clients, students, and volunteers. Personnel policies should address all aspects of HIV in the workplace, protect against social and economic discrimination, reflect the most current scientific and epidemiological knowledge, and incorporate sound principles of supervision and management. (Approved, September 1991).

HIV Testing/Confidentiality

AIDS Testing and ANA Policy, 1987

This policy was updated and incorporated into the 1991 "Position Statement on HIV Testing."

Serologic Testing of Health Care Workers for Human Immunodeficiency Virus Antibody, 1988

This policy was updated and incorporated into the 1991 "Position Statement on HIV Testing."

HIV Testing, 1991

ANA opposes perpetuation of the myth that mandatory testing and mandatory disclosure of the HIV status of patients and/or nurses is a method of preventing the transmission of HIV disease, and therefore does not advocate mandatory testing or mandatory disclosure of HIV status. ANA supports the availability of voluntary anonymous or confidential HIV testing that is conducted with informed consent, and pre- and post-test counseling. ANA continues to support education regarding the transmission of HIV/AIDS, and the use and monitoring of universal precautions to prevent HIV/AIDS transmission. (Approved, September 1991.)

Ethical Responsibility

The HIV-Infected Nurse, Ethical Obligations and Disclosure, 1992

The HIV-infected nurse is bound by the same precepts for practice as found in the *Code for Nurses*. The first duty is to protect the patient. Nurses who know that they have a transmissible bloodborne infection should voluntarily avoid exposure-prone invasive procedures that have been epidemiologically linked to HIV or other bloodborne infection transmission. The nurse has a duty to report exposure of a patient to bloodborne infection. Support and protection of the nurse with a seropositive status has been a long-standing position of ANA. The association supports the confidentiality of all information about the HIV-infected nurse. (Approved, December 1992.)

Guidelines for Disclosure to a Known Third Party About Possible HIV Infection, 1991

ANA supports the availability of voluntary and confidential partner notification services for HIV-positive individuals. ANA also endorses the concept of an ethical responsibility to disclose otherwise confidential information about probable HIV exposure when the patient fails to uphold his or her duty to protect others by preventing transmission of the infecting agent, but only when specific criteria have been met and documented. Partner notification should only be undertaken by a nurse or health care worker who is skilled in the biological and psychosocial aspects of HIV infection. (Approved, April 1991.)

Support for Confidential Notification Services, 1991

ANA supports voluntary confidential or anonymous HIV testing with pre- and post-test counseling, as well as the availability of voluntary and confidential partner notification services for HIV-positive individuals. Counseling should include information to prevent further transmission of the disease, and encouragement to personally inform a sex or needle-sharing partner of probable exposure to HIV. (Approved, April 1991).

Education

HIV Infection and Nursing Students, 1992

ANA supports comprehensive education regarding HIV/AIDS for all nursing students. Nursing curricula should include HIV/AIDS infection content, including treatment, transmission, mechanisms for protection while delivering care to persons with HIV/AIDS infection and hepatitis B (HBV) infection, and instruction in universal precautions and occupational safety and health issues. ANA believes that the HBV vaccine should be a required component of each nursing student's preclinical evaluation. Schools of nursing should develop a mechanism for disability coverage for students who contract HIV or HBV infection through exposure in the clinical setting, and nursing students should be assured of clinical setting protections consistent with those for employees covered under the Occupational Safety and Health Act. (Approved, April 1992.)

Curriculum Content for Nursing Care of AIDS Patients, 1988

This position statement was updated in 1992 by the "Position Statement on HIV Infection and Nursing Students."

B

HIV/AIDS *Resources*

AIDS Action Committee
131 Clarendon Street
Boston, MA 02116
617-437-6200

AIDS Action Council
1875 Connecticut Avenue, NW/Suite 700
Washington, DC 20009
202-986-1300

AIDS Virus Education and Research Institute (AVERI)
P.O. Box 31562
San Francisco, CA 94131
415-239-5200

American Foundation for AIDS Research (AMFAR)
733 Third Avenue, 12th Floor
New York, NY 10017
212-764-2060
   or
5900 Wilshire Boulevard/23rd Floor/
   East Satellite
Los Angeles, CA 90036-5032
213-857-5900

American Hospital Association Services Inc.
P.O. Box 92683
Chicago, IL 60675-2683
312-280-6000
800-242-2626

American Red Cross
National Headquarters/AIDS Education Office
431 18th Street, NW
Washington, DC 20006
202-737-8300

Centers for Disease Control and Prevention (CDC)
AIDS Office
2600 Executive Park Drive
Atlanta, GA 30329
404-639-3311 (switchboard)

CDC National AIDS Clearinghouse
P.O. Box 6003
Rockville, MD 20849-6003
800-458-5231

CDC National AIDS Hot Line
1600 Clifton Road/Building 1/Room B-63
Atlanta, GA 30333
800-342-AIDS

Computerized AIDS Information Network (CAIN)
P.O. Box 6182
San Francisco, CA 94101
415-864-4376

Gay Men's Health Crisis, Inc.
129 W. 20th Street
New York, NY 10011
212-807-7035
212-807-6655 (Hot Line)

Health Education Resources Organization
101 W. Read Street/Suite 825
Baltimore, MD 21201
410-685-1180
800-376-HERO
410-545-4774 (Hot Line)

Health Resources and Services Administration (HRSA)
Parklawn Building
5600 Fishers Lane/Room 7455
Rockville, MD 20857
Contact: Acting Chief/Division of AIDS
   Services/Room 9-13
301-443-6746

Hemophilia-AIDS Information Network (HANDI)
800-42-HANDI

Institute for Disease Prevention in the Workplace
4 Madison Place
Albany, NY 12202
518-456-1854

LAMBDA Legal Defense and Education Fund
666 Broadway/12th Floor
New York, NY 10012
212-995-8585
(9:30 a.m. to 5:30 p.m. weekdays)

National Association of People with AIDS
1413 K Street, NW/8th Floor
Washington, DC 20005
202-898-0414

National Center for Health Education
72 Spring Street, Suite 208
New York, NY 10012
212-334-9470

National Gay and Lesbian Task Force
1734 14th Street, NW
Washington, DC 20009
202-332-6483

National Leadership Coalition on AIDS
1730 M Street, NW/Suite 905
Washington, DC 20036
202-429-0930

National Lesbian and Gay Health Foundation
1407 S Street, NW
Washington, DC 20009
202-797-3708

Occupational Safety and Health Administration
U.S. Department of Labor
200 Constitution Avenue, NW/Room 725H
Washington, DC 20201
202-219-8148

Office of National AIDS Policy
Executive Office of the President
750 17th Street, NW/Suite 1060
Washington, DC 20503
202-632-1090

San Francisco AIDS Foundation
P.O. Box 426182
San Francisco, CA 94101
415-864-4376

United States Conference of Mayors
1620 I Street, NW/Suite 400
Washington, DC 20006
202-293-7330
(produces a directory of local AIDS-related services)

U.S. Public Health Service
Public Affairs Office
200 Independence Avenue, SW/
   Room 719H
Washington, DC 20201
202-690-6867

C

Definitions for
HIV/AIDS

The following represents the definition(s) currently being used to define HIV infection and AIDS in adolescents, adults, and the pediatric setting, from the CDC supplement entitled, *Revised Classification System for HIV Infection: An Expanded Surveillance Case Definition for AIDS among Adolescents and Adults* (1992). This supplement provides the current definitions and should be referred to for specific details.

In addition to adding three more clinical conditions, the revised classification system expanded the AIDS surveillance case definitions to include all HIV-infected persons who have less than 200 DCy T-lymphocytes (per microliter of blood), or a DCy + T-lymphocyte percentage of total lymphocytes of less than 14. The following list provides the 23 clinical conditions as published in 1987 plus the three previously noted additions which when diagnosed in an HIV-infected person equal meeting the case definition of AIDS.

HIV Infection, Adolescents > 13 Years and Adults

The criteria for HIV infection for persons 13 years of age and older include: a) repeatedly reactive screening tests for HIV antibody (e.g., enzyme immunoassay) with specific antibody identified by the use of supplemental tests (e.g., Western blot, immunofluorescence assay); b) direct identification of virus in host tissues by virus isolation; c) HIV antigen detection; or, d) a positive result on any other highly specific licensed test for HIV.

Consistent with the 1993 revised classification system, the CDC has also expanded the AIDS *surveillance case definition* to include all HIV-infected persons who have less than 200 CD4 + T-lymphocytes (per microliter of blood), or a CD4+ T-lymphocyte percentage of total lymphocytes of less than 14. This expansion also includes the addition of three clinical conditions—pulmonary tuberculosis, recurrent pneumonia, and invasive cervical cancer—and retains the 23 clinical conditions in the AIDS surveillance case definition published in 1987. It is to be used by all states for AIDS case reporting.

Clinical Conditions

1. Candidiasis of the esophagus, trachea, bronchi, or lungs
2. Cryptococcosis, extrapulmonary
3. Cryptosporidiosis with diarrhea persisting > 1 month
4. Cytomegalovirus disease of an organ other than liver, spleen, or lymph nodes in a patient > 1 month of age
5. Herpes simplex virus infection causing a mucocutaneous ulcer that persists longer than 1 month; or bronchitis, pneumonitis, or esophagitis for any duration affecting a patient > 1 month of age
6. Kaposi's sarcoma affecting a patient < 60 years of age
7. Lymphoma of the brain (primary) affecting a patient < 60 years of age
8. Lymphoid interstitial pneumonia and/or pulmonary lymphoid hyperplasia (LIP/PLH) complex affecting a child < 13 years of age)
9. Mycobacterium avium complex or M. kansasii disease, disseminated (at a site other than or in addition to lungs, skin, or cervical or hilar lymph nodes)
10. Pneumocystis carinii pneumonia
11. Progressive multifocal leukoencephalopathy
12. Toxoplasmosis of the brain affecting a patient > 1 month of age
13. Bacterial infections, multiple or recurrent (any combination of at least two within a two-year period), of the following types affecting a child < 13 years of age: septicemia, pneumonia,

meningitis, bone or joint infection, or abscess of an internal organ or body cavity (excluding otitis media or superficial skin or mucosal abscesses), caused by Hemophilus, Streptococcus (including pneumococcus), or other pyogenic bacteria

14. Coccidioidomycosis, disseminated (at a site other than or in addition to lungs or cervical or hilar lymph nodes)
15. HIV encephalopathy (also called "HIV dementia," "AIDS dementia," or "subacute encephalitis due to HIV")
16. Histoplasmosis, disseminated (at a site other than or in addition to lungs or cervical or hilar lymph nodes)
17. Isosporiasis with diarrhea persisting > 1 month
18. Kaposi's sarcoma at any age
19. Lymphoma of the brain (primary) at any age
20. Other non-Hodgkin's lymphoma of B-cell or unknown immunologic phenotype and the following histologic types:
    a. Small noncleaved lymphoma (either Burkitt or non-Burkitt type)
    b. Immunoblastic sarcoma (equivalent to any of the following, although not necessarily all in combination: immunoblastic lymphoma, large-cell diffuse histiocytic lymphoma, diffuse undifferentiated lymphoma, or high-grade lymphoma)
    Note: Lymphomas are not included here if they are of T-cell immunologic phenotype or their histologic type is not described, or is described as "lymphocytic," "lymphoblastic," "small cleaved," or "plasmacytoid lymphocytic."
21. Any mycobacterial disease caused by mycobacteria other than M. *tuberculosis*, disseminated (at a site other than or in addition to lungs, skin, cervical, or hilar lymph nodes)
22. Salmonella (nontyphoid) septicemia, recurrent
23. HIV wasting syndrome (emaciation, "slim disease)"
*24. Disease caused by M. *tuberculosis*
*25. Recurrent pneumonia (two or more episodes within a one-year period)
*26. Invasive cervical cancer
Indicates 1993 additions

HIV Infection in Children < 13 Years

Application of the definition for children differs from that for adults in two ways. First, multiple or recurrent serious bacterial infections and lymphoid interstitial pneumonia/pulmonary lymphoid hyperplasia are accepted as indicative of AIDS among children but not among adults. Second, for children less than 15 months of age whose mothers are thought to have had HIV infection during the child's perinatal period, the laboratory criteria for HIV infection are more stringent since the presence of HIV antibody in the child is, by itself, insufficient evidence for HIV infection because of the persistence of the passively acquired maternal antibodies less than 15 months after birth.

Classification System

CLASS PEDIATRIC-0	INDETERMINATE INFECTION	

1. Newborn < 15 months

2. Perinatally exposed infants < 15 months of age who have antibodies to HIV

CLASS PEDIATRIC-1	ASYMPTOMATIC INFECTION	

1. Subclass A: Normal immune function

2. Subclass B: Abnormal immune function

3. Subclass C: Immune function not tested

CLASS PEDIATRIC-2	SYMPTOMATIC INFECTION	

1. Subclass A: Non-specific findings

2. Subclass B: Progressive neurologic disease

3. Subclass C: Lymphoid interstitial pneumonitis

4. Subclass D: Secondary infectious diseases

    Category D-1: Specified secondary infectious diseases listed in the CDC surveillance definition for AIDS

    Category D-2: Recurrent serious bacterial infections

    Category D-3: Other specified secondary infectious diseases

5. Subclass E: Secondary cancers

    Category E-1: Specified secondary cancers listed in the CDC surveillance definition for AIDS

    Category E-2: Other cancers possibly secondary to HIV infection

6. Subclass F: Other diseases possibly due to HIV infection

For more details, contact the local AIDS Surveillance Office or the Centers for Disease Control and Prevention.

D

Universal Precautions

The Centers for Disease Control and Prevention have developed the strategy of "universal blood and body fluid precautions" to address concerns regarding the transmission of HIV and other bloodborne pathogens in the health care setting. The concept, now referred to simply as "universal precautions," stresses that all patients should be assumed to be infectious for HIV and other bloodborne pathogens (Centers for Disease Control 1989).

In hospitals and other health care settings, universal precautions should be followed when workers are exposed to blood and other body fluids, including semen, vaginal secretions, cerebrospinal fluid, synovial fluid, pleural fluid, pericardial fluid, peritoneal fluid, amniotic fluid, saliva in dental procedures, any body fluid visibly contaminated with blood, and all body fluids in situations where it is difficult or impossible to differentiate between body fluids (Occupational Safety and Health Administration 1992).

Since transmission has not been documented from exposure to feces, nasal secretions, sputum, sweat, tears, urine, or vomitus, universal precautions do not apply to these fluids (Centers for Disease Control 1989).

An occupational exposure is defined as contact with blood or other body fluids to which universal precautions apply through percutaneous inoculation or contact with an open wound, non-intact skin, or mucous membrane during the performance of normal job duties (Centers for Disease Control 1989).

Preventive measures include engineering and work practice controls and personal protective equipment. Each work setting should have a set of specific precautions and procedures appropriate to that setting. The following is a list of suggested general guidelines that apply to most health care situations:

1. Handle the blood and body fluids of all patients as potentially infectious.
2. Wear gloves for potential contact with blood or body fluids.
3. Wash hands after contact with blood or body fluids, including the handling of specimens, and when gloves are removed.
4. Wear gowns when splash with blood or body fluids is anticipated (e.g., in labor and delivery, trauma, and so on).
5. Wear protective eye wear and a mask if splatter with blood or body fluids is possible (e.g., when irrigating wounds, emptying containers, during relevant surgical procedures).
6. Used syringes and sharp objects (e.g., scalpels, lancets) should be discarded in appropriate containers as close to the point of use as possible.
7. If the procedure or condition warrants recapping, a one-handed scoop method or recapping device should be used.
8. Handle all linen soiled with blood and/or body secretions as infectious, wear gloves, and place in designated receptacles.
9. Process all laboratory specimens as potentially infectious.
10. Place resuscitation equipment where respiratory arrest is predictable.
11. Use disposal procedures appropriate to the equipment or materials being used, in accordance with CDC recommendations.
12. Reusable equipment (e.g., instruments) should be placed in appropriate containers for transport for cleaning and/or sterilization.

Universal precautions as defined by the CDC only protect against bloodborne pathogens, which leaves the need in a health care setting for additional infection precautions against other types of organisms. An alternative system of infection precautions has been proposed using the concept of a broad strategy that would serve the dual purpose of reducing cross-transmission risks to patients, while also protecting health care workers from microorganisms harbored by patients. This concept, termed *body substance isolation* (BSI), focuses on isolating all body substances from the hands of the health care worker, primarily by the appropriate use of gloves (Jackson 1992b).

All patients, including those infected with HIV, should be assessed for airborne transmittable infections (e.g., pulmonary TB, influenza) and, if so indicated, handled according to the institutional policies based on CDC guidelines.

The Standard on Occupational Exposure to Bloodborne Pathogens

E

(Occupational Safety and Health Administration, December 6, 1991)

Hospitals and other health care employers with one or more employees are required to:

- develop an exposure control plan that includes identification of employees with potential for occupational exposure;
- train all identified employees on occupational risks and methods to reduce risk;
- provide voluntary hepatitis B vaccines at no cost to identified employees;
- maintain records of employee training and medical evaluations;
- use warning labels and signs to identify hazards;
- implement methods to comply with provisions for worker protection, including universal precautions and the safe handling of sharps, specimens, contaminated laundry, and regulated waste;
- provide medical evaluation and treatment after exposure incidents;
- provide personal protective clothing and equipment;
- ensure employees are compliant;
- institute additional precautions for HIV and HBV research and production facilities, if applicable; and,
- evaluate the effectiveness of current safety technology.

Source: Copies of the full document, Title 29 Code of Federal Regulations, Part 1910.1030, or an overview of the contents can be obtained from the regional offices of OSHA.

F

The Americans with Disabilities Act

The Americans with Disabilities Act of 1990 (ADA) protects people with disabilities from discrimination in the areas of employment, public accommodations offered by private entities, and state and local government services, extending the limited protections afforded by the Rehabilitation Act of 1973. Not only are persons with HIV infection and disease covered by the act, but so are people who are regarded as being infected with HIV and people who are in close association with persons with HIV/AIDS. It is specifically the issue of HIV infection that is covered by the act, not other possible associated factors, such as being gay or being an injection drug user.

All nurses should be familiar with the different provisions of the ADA. Nurses who are discriminated against in the workplace because of a disability or perceived disability may be protected by Title I of the ADA. Further, it is important that staff nurses as well as nurse administrators be aware of the employment provisions, to ensure that appropriate policies are implemented by the employer in the workplace.

In addition, nurses should be aware of the different titles of the ADA so that they may advocate for their clients who are covered under its provisions. Finally, the nurse or other health care professional who refuses treatment to patients may be liable under the ADA. As the law is still developing—with its exact parameters refined and clarified as cases are resolved in court—different aspects of the act and its enforcement are still unknown.

In terms of workplace discrimination, the ADA covers employers of 15 or more employees. It prohibits state and local governments from discriminating against qualified individuals with disabilities in the provision of services or benefits, or in the use of government facilities otherwise available to the public. Finally, it prohibits private entities offering public accommodations from denying access or services to an individual with a disability on the basis of the disability, unless doing so would cause undue hardship. Public accommodations include physician's offices, hospitals, schools, pharmacies, hotels, and other public services (AIDS Action Council 1993).

The ADA provides protection from discrimination in the workplace for persons who, "with or without reasonable accommodation, can perform the essential functions of the employment position that such individual holds or desires." The concept of "reasonable accommodation" has already been defined under the 1973 Rehabilitation Act as modifications or adjustments to the job environment that enable the person to be qualified to perform the job, without undue hardship (i.e., resulting in significant difficulty or expense) for the employer, taking into account factors such as the size of the business and the cost of the accommodation (Feldblum 1992). An important point for persons with HIV infection is that if the person is qualified at the time of the employment decision, he or she cannot be rejected on the basis of possible disability or increased disability in the future.

An employer may not require an applicant for a job to submit to a medical examination or answer medical inquiries before a conditional job offer has been made. However, the employer may routinely require all job applicants for a specific job category to submit to a physical exam or blood testing (including HIV testing) after a conditional job offer has been made. The results must be kept strictly confidential and must not be used as the basis for withdrawing the conditional job offer unless the results indicate that the applicant is not qualified to perform the essential functions of the job (Feldblum 1992).

Recommendations on Management of Occupational Exposure to HIV

G

(Centers for Disease Control, January 26, 1990)

Definition of Occupational Exposure

The Centers for Disease Control and Prevention have defined an occupational exposure as "a percutaneous injury (e.g., a needle stick or cut with a sharp object), contact of mucous membranes, or contact with blood, tissues, or other body fluids to which universal precautions apply" (Centers for Disease Control 1990b).

Management after Possible Occupational Exposure to HIV

The CDC recommends that employers of health care workers should make available a system for promptly initiating evaluation, counseling, and follow-up after a reported occupational exposure that may place the worker at risk for acquiring HIV infection. Workers should be educated to report exposures immediately after they occur, in order to obtain hepatitis B prophylaxis and other possible interventions immediately.

Workers considered at risk for occupational exposure to blood-borne pathogens should be taught the principles of post-exposure management as part of job orientation and ongoing job training. In particular, they should be trained to immediately wash any remaining fluid off or out of the injured area, to flush mucous membranes, and to wash skin with running water and soap. After an exposure occurs, the employee should have immediate access to a staff person trained in post-exposure management, including counseling, and the appropriate interventions should be initiated.

The circumstances of the exposure should be recorded in the worker's confidential medical record. Information should include date and time of exposure; job duty being performed; details of exposure, including amount and type of fluid or material, and severity of exposure; description of source of exposure, including, if known, whether the source material contained HIV or HBV; and details about interventions initiated with the worker, including counseling, post-exposure management, and follow-up.

If the exposed worker has not been vaccinated against hepatitis B, a course of vaccine should be offered. In addition, if the source patient or material is evaluated and found to be positive for hepatitis B surface antigen, hepatitis B immunoglobulin may also be indicated.

In addition, the source individual should be informed of the incident and, if consent is obtained, tested for serologic evidence of HIV infection. If consent cannot be obtained (e.g., the patient is unconscious or refuses), policies should be developed for testing source individuals in compliance with applicable state and local laws. *Confidentiality of the source individual should be maintained at all times.*

If the source individual is known to be HIV-positive or have AIDS, or refuses testing, the worker should be evaluated clinically and serologically for evidence of HIV infection as soon as possible after the exposure. If the worker is seropositive, this is an indication that he or she was already infected prior to the occupational incident. If the worker is seronegative, he or she should be retested periodically for a minimum of six months post-exposure to determine whether HIV infection has occurred.

The worker should be advised to report and seek medical evaluation for any acute illness that occurs during the follow-up period. During the follow-up period, the exposed worker should follow Public Health Service recommendations for preventing transmission of HIV. These recommendations include refraining from blood, semen, or organ donation; and abstaining from, or using measures to prevent HIV transmission during, sexual contact. In addition, in countries such as the United States where safe and effective alternatives to breast-feeding are available, exposed women should not breastfeed infants. *During all phases of follow-up, confidentiality of the worker should be protected.*

If the source individual is HIV-negative and has no clinical manifestations of AIDS or HIV infection, no further HIV follow-up of the exposed worker is necessary unless epidemiologic evidence suggests that the source individual may have recently been exposed to HIV or if testing is desired by the worker or recommended by the health care provider. In these instances, the guidelines should be followed as described above. If the source individual cannot be identified, decisions regarding appropriate follow-up should be individualized, based on factors such as whether potential sources are likely to include a person at increased risk of HIV infection.

The employer should make serologic testing available to all workers who are concerned about possible infection with HIV through an occupational exposure. Appropriate psychological counseling may be indicated as well.

Consideration of Zidovudine Prophylaxis

The CDC discusses the additional option of offering zidovudine to exposed workers as a possible means of prophylaxis from seroconverting to HIV. The use of zidovudine for post-exposure prophylaxis is based on the speculation that the antiviral properties of the drug may inhibit replication in the exposed health care worker.

The efficacy of zidovudine prophylaxis has not been demonstrated, either in animal studies (Ruprecht et al. 1986; Tavares et al. 1987) or in prospective monitoring of occupationally exposed health care workers who have opted to take zidovudine. However, given the low probability of seroconversion in the first place, it is extremely difficult to document whether zidovudine prophylaxis contributes protection to the exposed health care worker. (In the CDC surveillance study, four out of 1,103 enrolled workers with percutaneous exposure to HIV-infected blood seroconverted, resulting in an HIV seroconversion rate of 0.35 percent for percutaneous exposure. No enrolled workers with mucous membrane or skin contact seroconverted [Tokars et al. 1993]). What cannot be determined is whether additional seroconversions would have occurred if the participants had not completed the course of prophylactic medication.

From October 1988 through June 1992, 31 percent to 43 percent of the health care workers enrolled in the CDC surveillance study of HIV occupational exposure opted to use zidovudine after exposure. Despite using zidovudine after exposure, one worker became infected with a strain of HIV that apparently was sensitive to zidovudine. Three-quarters of the workers taking zidovudine complained of adverse symptoms. Nearly one-third of the health care workers did not complete the planned courses of zidovudine because of the adverse symptoms (Tokars 1993).

An expert in HIV occupational exposure states that the decision to use zidovudine after exposure is very individual and personal. Exposed health care workers who are considering treatment with zidovudine should be fully informed that its value for prophylaxis is unproven to date (Gerberding 1993).

REFERENCES

AIDS Action Council. 1993. *The Americans with Disabilities Act*. The Author: Washington, DC.

American Hospital Association. 1992. *OSHA's final bloodborne pathogens standard: A special briefing*. Chicago: American Hospital Association.

American Nurses Association. 1985. *Code for nurses with interpretive statements*. Kansas City, Mo.: American Nurses Association.

————. 1988. *Nursing and HIV: A response to the problem*. Kansas City, Mo.: American Nurses Association.

————. 1991. *Standards of clinical nursing practice*. Kansas City, Mo.: American Nurses Association.

————. 1993. *Compendium of HIV/AIDS positions, policies and documents*. Washington, DC: American Nurses Publishing.

Bartlett, J.G. 1988. Testing for HIV infection: Recommendations for surgeons. *American College of Surgeons Bulletin* 73(3):4-10.

Bastian, L.; Bennett, C.L.; Adams, J.; Waskin, H.; Divine, G.; and Edlin, R. 1993. Differences between men and women with HIV-related PCP: Experience from 3,070 cases in New York City in 1987. *Journal of Acquired Immune Deficiency Syndrome* 6(6):617-623.

Becker, M.H., and Joseph, J.G. 1988. AIDS and behavioral change to reduce risk: A review. *American Journal of Public Health* Apr 78(4):394-410.

Bennett, J. 1987. Nurses talk about the challenge of AIDS. *American Journal of Nursing* 77(9):1151-1155.

Boland, M.G. and Conviser, R. 1992. Nursing care of the child. In *HIV/AIDS: A guide to nursing care*, 2nd ed., eds. J.H. Flaskerud and P. Ungvarski, pp 199-238. Philadelphia: W.B. Saunders.

Brown, B.L. and Brown, J.W. 1988. The Third International Conference on AIDS: Risk of AIDS in health care workers. *Nursing Management* 19(3):33-35.

————. 1981a. Kaposi's sarcoma, pneumocystis pneumonia among homosexual men—NYC and California. *Morbidity and Mortality Weekly Report* 30:305-308.

————. 1981b. Pneumocystis pneumonia—Los Angeles. *Morbidity and Mortality Weekly Report* 30:250-252.

————. 1984. Acquired immunodeficiency syndrome (AIDS)—United States. *Morbidity and Mortality Weekly Report* 32(49):688-691.

————. 1985. Education and foster care of children infected with human T-lymphotropic virus type III/lymphadenopathy-associated virus. *Morbidity and Mortality Weekly Report* 34(34):517-520.

————. 1987a. Classification system for HIV infection in children under 13 years of age. *Morbidity and Mortality Weekly Report* 36(15):225-230, 235.

————. 1987b. HIV infection in the U.S. *Morbidity and Mortality Weekly Report* 36(49):801-804.

————. 1987c. Recommendations for prevention of HIV transmission in health care settings. *Morbidity and Mortality Weekly Report* 36(2S):81-118.

————. 1989. Guidelines for prevention of transmission of HIV and hepatitis B virus to health-care and public safety workers. *Morbidity and Mortality Weekly Report* 38(S-6):1-37.

————. 1990a. Guidelines for preventing the transmission of tuberculosis in health-care settings, with special focus on HIV-related issues. *Morbidity and Mortality Weekly Report* 39(RR-17):81-129.

————. 1990b. Management of occupational exposure to HIV, including considerations regarding zidovudine post-exposure use. *Morbidity and Mortality Weekly Report* 39(RR-1):81-114.

————. 1991a. Drug use and sexual behaviors among sex partners of injection-drug users: United States, June 1981—December 1991. *Morbidity and Mortality Weekly Report* 40(49):855-860.

————. 1991b. Mortality attributable to HIV infection/AIDS—United States, 1981-1990. *Morbidity and Mortality Weekly Report* 40(3):41-44.

————. 1991c. Nosocomial transmission of multidrug-resistant tuberculosis among HIV-infected persons—Florida and New York, 1988-1991. *Morbidity and Mortality Weekly Report* 40:585-591.

————. 1991d. Update: Transmission of HIV infection during an invasive dental procedure—Florida. *Morbidity and Mortality Weekly Report* 40(2):21-33.

————. 1992. Revised classification system for HIV infection: An expanded surveillance case definition for AIDS among adolescents and adults. *Morbidity and Mortality Weekly Report* 41(RR-17):1-19.

————. 1993a. HIV/AIDS *Surveillance Report*, second-quarter edition, July 1993. 5(2):1-19.

————. 1993b. HIV/AIDS *Surveillance Report*, year-end edition, Feb. 1993:1-23.

————. 1993c. Update: AIDS—United States, 1992. *Morbidity and Mortality Weekly Report* 42(28):547-557.

————. 1993d. Update: Mortality attributable to HIV infection/AIDS among persons aged 25-44 years—United States, 1990 and 1991. *Morbidity and Mortality Weekly Report* 42(25):481-486.

References

Coyle, S.L.; Boruch, R.F.; and Turner, C.F., eds. 1991. *Evaluating AIDS prevention programs.* Washington, DC: National Academy Press.

Curtis, J.R. and Patrick, D.L. 1993. Race and survival time with AIDS: A synthesis of the literature. *American Journal of Public Health* 83(10):1425-1428.

Durham, J.D. 1991. Ethical and legal dimensions. In *The person with AIDS: Nursing perspectives*, eds. J.D. Durham and F.L. Cohen, pp 361-387. New York: Springer.

Feldblum, R. 1992. Workplace issues: HIV and discrimination. In *AIDS agenda: Emerging issues in civil rights*, eds. N.D. Hunter and W.B. Rubenstein, Part III, p 271. New York: The New York Press.

Fife, D. and McAnaney, J. 1993. Private medical insurance among Philadelphia residents diagnosed with AIDS. *Journal of Acquired Immune Deficiency Syndrome* 6(5):512-517.

Fisher, J.D. and Misovich, S.J. 1990. Social influence and HIV-preventive behavior. In *Social influence processes and prevention*, eds. J. Edwards, R.S. Tindale, L. Heath, and E.J. Posevac, pp. 39-70. New York: Plenum.

Flaskerud, J.H. 1987. AIDS: Neuropsychiatric complications. *Journal of Psychosocial Nursing* 25(12):17-20.

Freudenberg, N. 1989. *Preventing AIDS: A guide to effective education for the prevention of HIV infection.* Washington, DC: American Public Health Association Press.

Gebbie, K. 1990. Current and future impact of HIV on nursing. In *Nursing and the HIV epidemic: A National action agenda*, eds. T.P. Phillips and D. Black. Washington, DC: U.S. Department of Health and Human Services.

Gerberding, J.L. 1986. Recommended infection control policies for patients with HIV infection. *New England Journal of Medicine* 315(24):1562-1564.

———. 1992. Needlestick prevention: New paradigms for research. *Infect. Control Hosp Epidemiol.* May 13(5):257-258.

———. 1993. Is antiretroviral treatment after percutaneous HIV exposure justified? *Annals of Internal Medicine* 118(12):979-980.

Gerberding, J.L.; Bryant-LeBlanc, C.E.; Nelson, K.; Moss, A.R.; Osmond, D.; Chambers, H.F.; Carlson, J.R.; Drew, W.L.; Levy, J.A., and Sande, M.A. 1987. Risk of transmitting the HIV, CMV, and hepatitis B virus to health care workers exposed to patients with AIDS and AIDS-related conditions. *Journal of Infectious Diseases* 156(1):1-8.

Gershon, R.M.; Vlahov, D.; and Nelson, K.E. 1990. HIV infection risk to nonhealth-care workers. *American Indian Hygiene Association Journal* 51(12):A807-809.

Hanson, D.L.; Horsburgh, C.R., Jr.; Fann, S.A.; Havlik, J.A.; and Thompson, S.E., III. 1993. Survival prognosis of HIV-infected patients. *Journal of Acquired Immune Deficiency Syndrome* 6(6):624-629.

Haverkos, H.W.; Gottlieb, M.S.; Killen, J.Y.; and Edelman, R. 1985. Classification of HTLVIII/LAV-related diseases. *Journal of Infectious Diseases* 152(5):1095.

Hein, K. 1992. Adolescents at risk for HIV infection. In *Adolescents and AIDS: A generation in jeopardy*, ed. J. DiClemente, p. 4. Newbury Park, Calif.: Sage Publications.

Hellinger, F.J. 1993. The lifetime cost of treating a person with HIV. *Journal of the American Medical Association* 270(4):474-478.

Henderson, D.K. Saah, H.J.; Zak, B.J.; Kaslow, R.A., 1986. Risk of nosocomial infection with human T-cell lymphotropic virus type III/lymphadenopathy-associated virus in a large cohort of intensively exposed health care workers. *Annals of Internal Medicine* 104(5):644-647.

Hendrik, J.C.; Medley, G.F.; van Griensven, G.J.P.; Coutinho, R.A.; Heisterkamp, S.H.; and van Druten, H.A.M. 1993. The treatment-free incubation period of AIDS in a cohort of homosexual men. *AIDS* 7(2):231-239.

Institute of Medicine. 1986. *Institute of Medicine report: Confronting AIDS directions*. Washington, DC: National Academy of Sciences Press.

Jackson, M.M. 1992a. Infection prevention and control. *Critical Care Nursing Clinics of North America* 4(3):401-409.

———. 1992b. *Information packet on the OSHA regulations on bloodborne pathogens*. San Diego: University of California at San Diego Medical Center.

Jackson, M.H. 1992. Health insurance: The battle over limits on coverage. In *AIDS agenda: Emerging issues in civil rights*, eds. N.D. Hunter and W.B. Rubenstein, Part II, p. 147. New York: The New York Press.

Jenna, J. 1987. Care for the caregiver. *Health Care Forum Journal* 30(6):23-26.

Jenna, J.K., and Mount, A.H. 1988. AIDS management: New models for care. *Healthcare Forum* 30(6), 18-22, 46-48.

Jonsen, R. and Stryker, J., eds. 1993. *The social impact of AIDS in the United States*. Washington, DC: National Academy Press.

Kalichman, S.C.; Kelly, J.A.; Hunter, T.L.; Murphy, D.A.; and Tyler, R. 1993. Culturally tailored HIV/AIDS risk-reduction messages targeted to African-American urban women: Impact on risk sensitization and risk reduction. *Journal of Consultation in Clinical Psychology* 61(2):291-295.

Keller, E. 1993. SSA releases new HIV regulations. Paper presented to the AIDS Legal Referral Panel, San Francisco.

Kelly, J.A.; St. Lawrence, J.S.; Diaz, Y.E.; Stevenson, Y.; Hauth, A.C.; Brasfield, T.; Kalichman, S.C.; Smith, J.E.; and Andrew, M.E. 1991. HIV risk behavior reduction following intervention with key opinion leaders of population: An experimental analysis. *American Journal of Public Health* 81(2):168-171.

Kramer, F.; Modilevsky, T.; et al. 1990. Delayed diagnosis of tuberculosis in patients with HIV infection. *American Journal of Medicine* 89:451-456.

Krasinski, K.; Borkowsky, W.; and Holzman, R.S. 1989. Prognosis of HIV infection in children and adolescents. *Pediatric Infectious Diseases Journal* 8(4):216-220.

Kraut, A. 1987. *AIDS counseling and HIV-antibody testing: A position paper*. Coalition for AIDS Prevention and Education of National Organizations Responding to AIDS.

Mann, J.; Tarantola, D.; and Netter, T., eds. 1992. *AIDS in the world*. Cambridge, Mass.: Harvard University Press.

McArthur, J.H. and McArthur, J.C. 1986. Neurological manifestations of AIDS. *Journal of Neuroscience Nursing* 18(5):242-249.

Moss, F. and Miles, H. 1987. AIDS and the geriatrician. *Journal of the American Geriatric Society* 35(5):460-464.

Moulton, J.; Sweet, D.; Gurbuz, G.; and Dilley, J.W. 1989. Do groups work? Evaluation of a group model. In J.W. Dilley, C. Pies, and M. Helquist, eds. *Face to face: A guide to* AIDS *counseling,* pp 94-101. San Francisco: The AIDS Health Project, University of California at San Francisco.

National Association of People with AIDS. 1992. HIV *in America: A profile of the challenges facing Americans living with* HIV. Washington, D.C.: National Association of People with AIDS.

National Commission on AIDS. 1992. *The challenge of* HIV/AIDS *in communities of color.* U.S. Government Printing Office: Washington, DC.

National Institute for Nursing Research. 1993. Setting nursing research priorities. Unpublished paper, Washington, DC

National Research Council. 1993. *The social impact of* AIDS *in the United States.* Washington, DC: National Academy Press.

Occupational Safety and Health Administration. 1992. *Occupational exposure to blood-borne pathogens.* Washington, DC: Occupational Safety and Health Administration, U.S. Department of Labor.

Pratt, R.D.; Hatch, R.; Dankner, W.M.; and Spector, S.A. 1993. Pediatric HIV infection in a low seroprevalence area. *Pediatric Infectious Disease Journal* 12(4):304-310.

Redfield, R.R.; Wright, D.C.; and Tramant, E.C. 1986. The Walter Reed staging classification of HTLV-III infection. *New England Journal of Medicine* 314(2):131-132.

Ruprecht, R.M.; O'Brien, L.G.; Rossoni, L.D.; and Nusinoff-Lehrman, S. 1986. Suppression of mouse viraemia and retroviral disease by 3'-azido-3'-deoxythymidine. *Nature* 323(6087):467-469.

Sabin, C.; Phillips, A.; Elford, J.; Griffiths, P.; Janossay, G.; and Lee, C. 1993. The progression of HIV disease in a hemophiliac cohort followed for 12 years. *British Journal of Hematology* 83(2):330-333.

Sedaka, S.B. 1986. Financial implications of AIDS. *Caring* 38(June):38-46.

Shacknai, D. 1992. Wealth = health: The public financing of AIDS care. In AIDS *agenda: Emerging issues in civil rights,* eds. N.D. Hunter and W.B. Rubenstein, Part II, p. 181. New York: The New York Press.

Sowell, R.L.; Gueldner, S.H.; Killeen, M.R.; Lowenstein, A.; Fuszard, B.; and Swansburg, R. 1992. Impact of case management on hospital charges of PWAs in Georgia. *Journal of the Association of Nurses in AIDS Care* 3(2):24-31.

Sutin, D.G.; Rose, D.N.; Mulvihill, M.; and Taylor, B. 1993. Survival of elderly patients with transfusion-related AIDS. *Journal of the American Geriatric Society* 41(3):214-216.

Tavares, L.; Roneker, C.; Johnston, K.; Nusinoff-Legrman, S.; and De Noronha, F. 1987. 3'-azido-3'-deoxythymidine in feline leukemia virus-infected cats: A model for therapy and prophylaxis of AIDS. *Cancer Research* 47(12):3190-3194.

Tokars, J.I.; Marcus, R.; Culver, D.H.; Schable, C.A.; Bell, M.; McKibben, P.S., Bandea, C.I. 1993. Surveillance of HIV infection and zidovudine use among health care workers after occupational exposure to HIV-infected blood. *Annals of Internal Medicine* 118(12):913-919.

Turner, B.J.; Denison, M.; Eppes, S.C.; Houchens, R.; Fanning, T.; and Markson, L.E. 1993. Survival experience of 789 children with AIDS. *Pediatric Infectious Disease Journal* 12(4):310-320.

U.S. Public Health Service. 1988. Report of the Second Public Health Service AIDS Prevention and Control Conference: Report of the workgroup on epidemiology and surveillance. *Public Health Reports* 103 suppl 1( ):10-18.

Valenti, W.M. 1992. *Early intervention in the management of* HIV. U.S.A.: Burroughs Wellcome Co.

von Reyn, F. and Mann, J. 1987. Global epidemiology. *Western Journal of Medicine* 147(6):694-701.

Wright, J.; Henry, S.B.; Holzemer, W.L.; and Falknor, P. 1993. Evaluation of community-based nurse case management activities for symptomatic HIV/AIDS clients. *Journal of the Association of Nurses in AIDS Care* 4(2):37-47.